AN ILLUSTRATED GUIDE TO
EVERYDAY EURYTHMY

Translated by Matthew Barton

Contributors: Manfred Christ, Kristian Schneider, Ulrike Schiener,
Juliane Sonntag, Barbara Tapfer, Annette Weißkircher, Michael Weißkircher
Photography: Frank Gottinger, Patricia Gapp
First published in German as *Eurythmie Therapie: Ein Übungsbuch*
by Futurum Verlag, Basel in 2016
First published in English by Floris Books in 2017

© 2016 Futurum Verlag, Basel
English version © Floris Books 2017

All rights reserved. No part of this publication may
be reproduced without the prior permission of
Floris Books, Edinburgh
www.florisbooks.co.uk
ISBN 978-178250-373-6
Printed in Poland

AN ILLUSTRATED GUIDE TO
EVERYDAY EURYTHMY

Barbara Tapfer
Annette Weißkircher

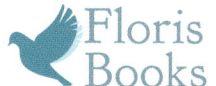
Floris Books

Contents

Introduction

Why is eurythmy important?	8
Length of treatment	9
Matching sound and form	9

Vowel Exercises

Getting started	14
A (ah) opening	17
E (eh) crossing	23
I (ee) reaching out from the heart space	33
O (oh) circular enclosing	41
U (oo) bringing together	47

Consonant Exercises

Getting started	57
B enveloping and protecting	59
P enveloping and drawing in	65
D gently descending	71
T inwardly radiating	77
F airborne intention	83
G calmly repelling	87
K energetically repelling	93

■ H broadening and freeing	97
■ L wavelike transformation	101
■ M supple sensing	107
■ N quickly withdrawing	121
■ R revolving	125
■ S enlivening and formative	131
■ Sh narrowly spiralling upward	139

Soul Exercises

■ A (ah) reverence	150
■ E (eh) love	152
■ U (oo) hope	154
■ Yes / no	156
■ Sympathy / antipathy	158

Resources

| Further reading | 160 |

Introduction

> Dance nurtures the liberated, resonant human being, with all his powers in balance.
>
> *St Augustine*

In eurythmy, musical tones and the different sounds of human speech are transformed into a system of distinct whole-body movements that correspond to the archetypal and universal sounds of music and speech. These gentle gestures can be practised as harmonising, therapeutic exercises that embody the formative power of language and make visible the invisible gestures inherent in speech.

Eurythmy was conceived in 1912 as a new mode of artistic expression. The therapeutic potential of this new form was soon recognised and has developed alongside artistic, performance-oriented eurythmy for nearly a century. Always in movement, never static, it is an *active* therapy that draws on the original power of human speech in order to stimulate an individual's innate ability to self-heal, working right into the organic functions of the human body.

Therapeutic eurythmists work in conjunction with a physician, and always in accordance with the patient's individual constitution. The basic four-year, full-time artistic eurythmy training program is offered in over twenty-five countries. Further training in therapeutic eurythmy is a three-year, part-time course resulting in a certificate from the Medical Section of the School of Spiritual Science in Dornach, Switzerland. Eurythmy therapy is available all over the world, but it is often the case that a lack of funding makes it difficult for those seeking therapy to obtain a complete course of treatment (ideally between twelve and fifteen sessions).

This book was created in response to that situation, and aims to offer support for both patients and therapists who may not be able to receive or provide a sufficient amount of individual therapy. It uses pictures and words to illustrate the basic speech-sound exercises and represents a first attempt to photographically record basic eurythmy therapy movements and patterns. These 'moving pictures' and step-by-step guidelines can offer support for patients who wish to continue practising on their own.

This project was the courageous initiative of Barbara Tapfer, a Masters student of eurythmy therapy at Alanus University, Germany. With the help of a committed team of professionals, she was able to bring this book – and the movements within – to life.

Readers who would like to learn more about eurythmy and its therapeutic potential, or who wish to look for an experienced therapist in their area, will find helpful resources at the end of the book.

Remember, this is just the beginning: many aspects and elements used in eurythmy therapy could not be included here, such as sequences of speech sounds, spatial forms, rhythms, body meditations, tone eurythmy therapy, eye eurythmy therapy or dental eurythmy therapy. For now, the gestures in this book provide a foundation for bringing living, healing relationships to the whole human being – body, soul and spirit.

Annette Weißkircher

Please note

The contents and exercises of this workbook were carefully researched, tested and discussed with experts. They can offer guidance and orientation for patients practising on their own, and serve as a reminder, but they are not a substitute for the work of a physician or eurythmy therapist, and are not intended as such. The authors and publisher are not liable where such use occurs.

Why is eurythmy important?

Human communication occurs above all through speech, which conveys not only information but also the inner soul experience. Infants feel their parents' love and protection not just through their words but also in the soft, empathic tones of their voices. In contrast, warnings of danger are signalled not only as 'pure information' but through a strong, sharp 'Stop!'.

When volume and tone accompany words, our inner feelings resonate through the whole body, but it doesn't stop there. Physical gestures give further life to our communication. We don't have to learn how to do it – non-verbal communication is innate – but we are doing it less and less.

It is believed that people once accompanied speech with much stronger and more expressive gestures than they do now. We still gesticulate today, of course, when animatedly telling a story, greeting a loved one or having a quarrel, our movements and facial expressions enhancing our message. Many people also continue to ascribe a primal power to specific words and actions – for instance in prayer or meditation, where we seek a positive, consciousness-enlarging effect from our movements and mantras.

But nowadays, humans spend much of their day communicating through written language, where gestures are redundant and words tend to become ever more schematic in quality. This reduction of language to its purely intellectual content has an effect on us, right into our physiology: when we do not engage physically with language, our metabolism is not sufficiently perfused with blood.

It has been clinically proven that those who speak with the full power of their breath and accompany their words with purposeful gestures have improved breathing capacity and blood circulation. A study conducted by Dirk Cysarz et al. in 2004 showed that the recitation of poetry had a positive effect on the heart. The test subjects felt livelier and more equable afterwards than they had beforehand. In fact, they felt a deep tranquillity and harmony, such as we usually only experience after recuperative sleep.

Therapeutic eurythmists aim to do a more specialised version of this for their patients: modifying specific speech gestures to suit each particular person's needs. For over eighty years, this form of anthroposophical treatment has been used in general and clinical practice, palliative care and rehabilitation for the treatment of acute, chronic or degenerative disorders of the nervous system, the cardiovascular system, the respiratory system, the metabolic system, and the musculoskeletal system. It is also used for eye disorders, dental misalignment, in psychosomatic medicine, psychiatry, and for childhood developmental disorders and disabilities.

Length of treatment

The length of a single treatment session is determined by the type of illness, the patient's age, and their state of health. A course of treatment usually involves one session a week for between 12 and 25 sessions. Each session is followed by a rest of about 15 minutes. Depending on medical indication, each session will last between 30 and 60 minutes.

Matching sound and form

In speech or singing, the whole range of the human body's movement is recapitulated in miniature in the fine, differentiated movements of the laryngeal muscles, the mouth and pharynx. Using special filming techniques, we can see evidence of the connection between these synchronous micro-movements with movement impulses in the rest of the body. The aim of eurythmy is to make these impulses visible.

Vowels sound forth through the chest and larynx, giving the voice its distinctive timbre and conveying the inner soul's expression. They are therefore expressed in eurythmy as gestures that imitate the position of the vocal cords and glottis during phonation.

Consonants are sculpted through the lips and the activity of the tongue with the teeth and the palate. In eurythmy, these small movements are changed into large, lively, shaping forms.

Eurythmy speech-sound gestures are thus differentiated, each sound conveying its own distinctive archetypal power: the formative force that underlies all nature's living, organic life. By turning words and single speech sounds into movement in eurythmy, the human body becomes an instrument.

As we piece sounds together through movement to form words, we may find that some words have characteristic affinities with their symbolic form or morphology. Neuroscientist Vilayanur Ramachandran, who teaches at the University of California in San Diego, wanted to show that sounds are linked to visual shapes. Half in jest, he drew two shapes on the board in front of an audience: one with rounded and the other with angular shapes, claiming that these formed part of the Martian alphabet:

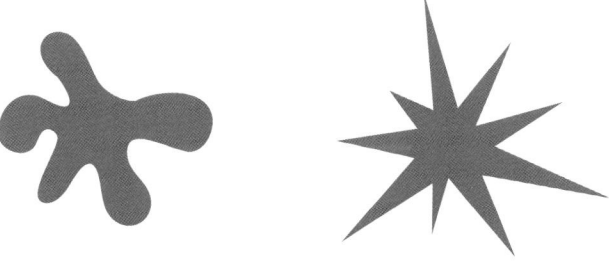

He asked his audience which word meant '*bouba*' and which word meant '*kiki*'. Amazingly, ninety-five per cent of participants felt that *bouba* accorded with the rounded form, whereas *kiki* would better suit the angular shape.

The 'Bouba-Kiki Effect' could be explained by a phenomenon called synaesthesia, in which different senses are connected in the brain. The sharp sounds of the word *kiki*, made by the tapping movements of palate and tongue in the mouth, imitate the sharp spikes of the symbol. Similarly, the soft contours of the *bouba* sound, and the movements of lips and tongues required to make it, reflect the gentle contour of the round, cloud-like form.

The same can be said for the movements belonging to these sounds in eurythmy. For B, a round, encompassing gesture is made, while the gesture for K is angular and sharp.

Introduction

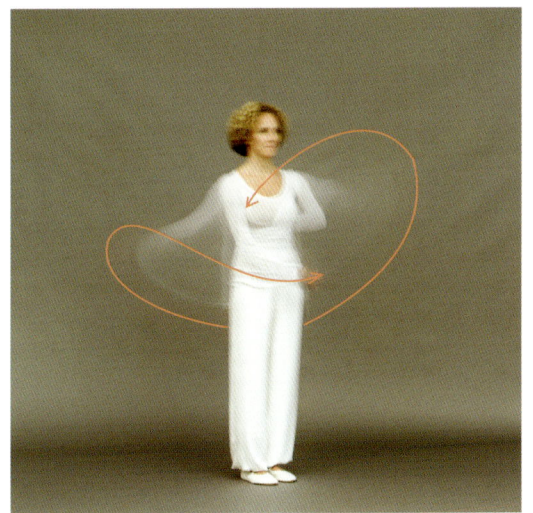

B

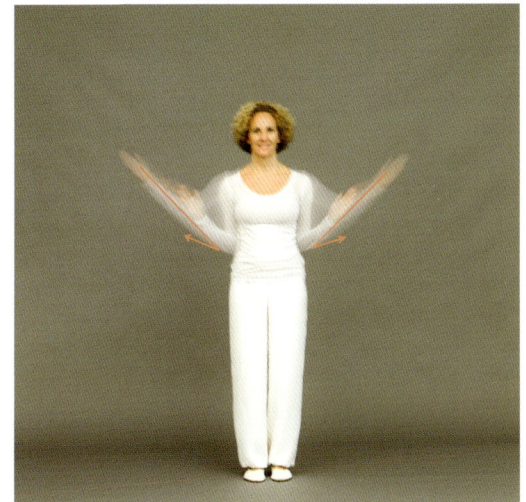

K

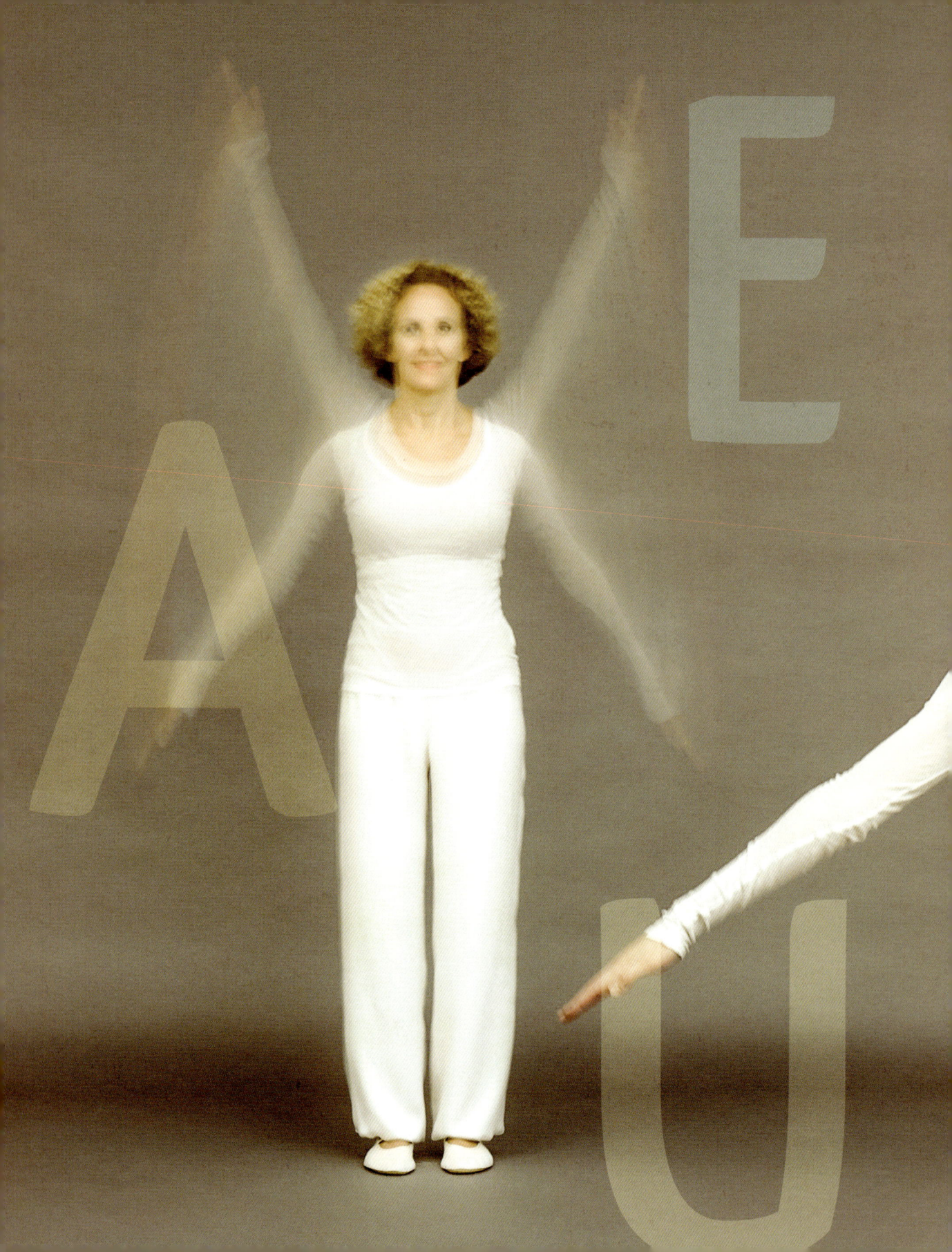

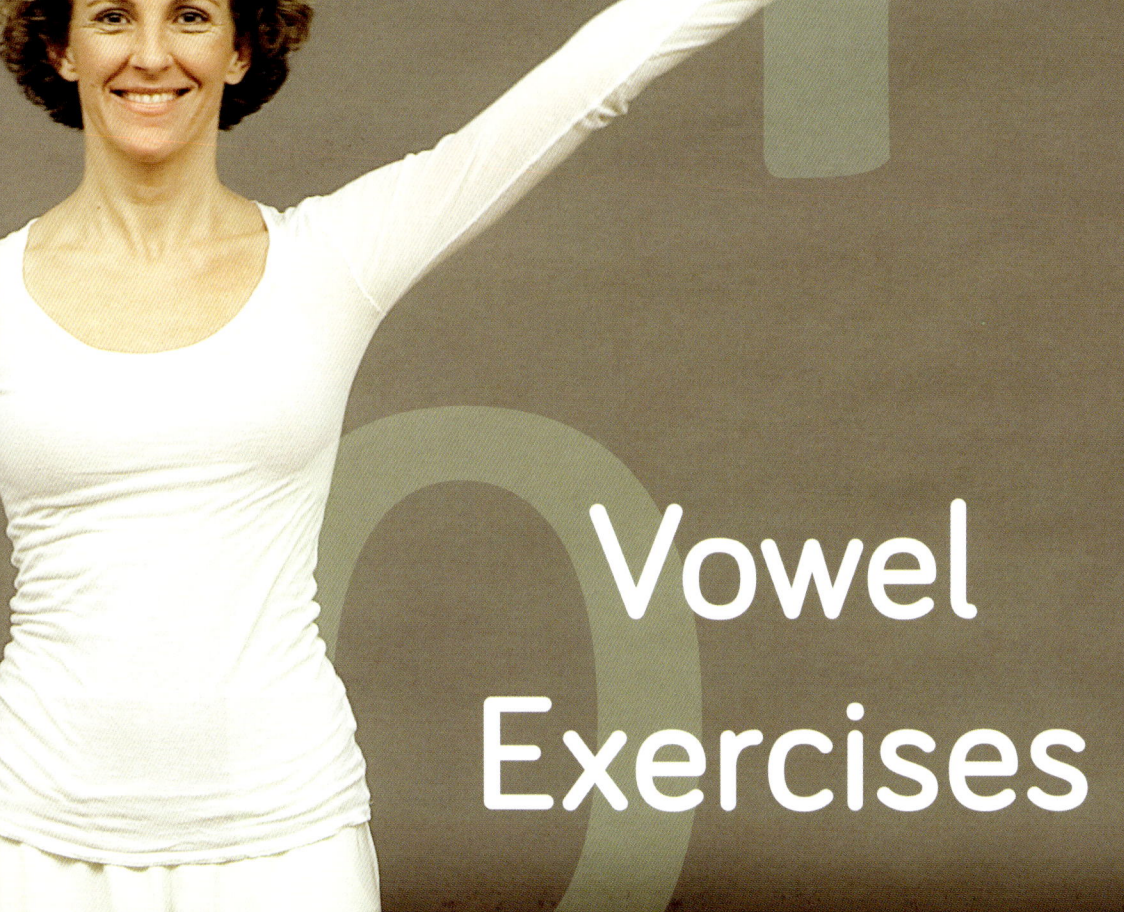

Vowel Exercises

Getting started

Every vowel exercise in eurythmy therapy has three stages:

1. Speaking or intoning the vowel
2. Moving arms, then legs, then arms again
3. Listening to the resonance of this sound and movement

1. Speaking

First, the vowel is spoken a few times (roughly three) on the outbreath.

2. Moving arms and legs in alternation

Each vowel varies slightly, but usually the gestures are performed slowly at first, with the arms starting above the head, moving downward in five to seven stages. After this has been repeated slowly, it should be performed rapidly with swinging arms.

The vowel is then formed the same number of times with the legs (either standing in place or with a little step between each gesture).

The arm movements are then repeated.

3. Resonance

Now we can:

- listen to the echo of the vowel;
- let it resonate within our soul;
- perceive what effect is felt in us;
- calmly observe anything that naturally occurs.

Soul mood and intention

Nowadays we are accustomed to doing one thing while thinking about another. It requires our full attention, however, to 'shape' the vowel sounds with movement. The more attention we can give to that moment in time, the more profound an effect this will have on our inner soul mood.

The following steps will help make vowel gestures more intentional as you try to sense your arms and legs right into their muscle tone:

- As you form the angle of an A (ah) gesture, experience the gesture's liberating, opening impetus.
- As you form the crossing E (eh) gesture, feel for a centring at the place where your arms intersect.
- As you form a reaching I (ee) gesture, sense a radiating drive, extending in two opposite directions.
- As you form an encircling O (oh) gesture, open yourself to an encompassing force.
- As you form an U (oo) gesture, sense its contracting impulse through the parallel orientation of your limbs.

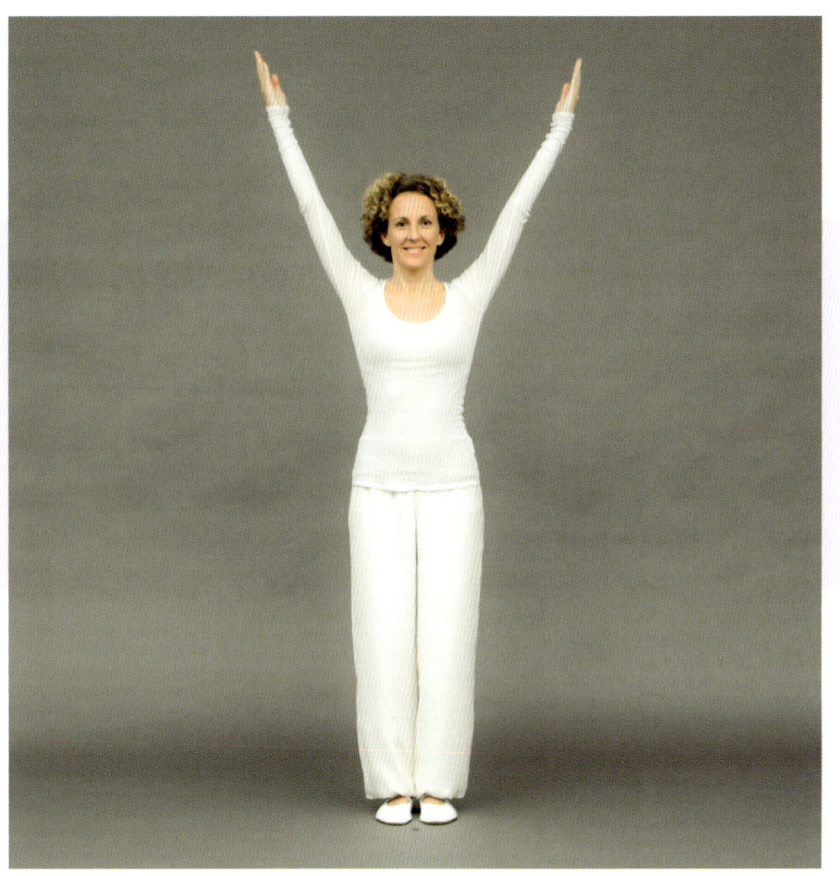
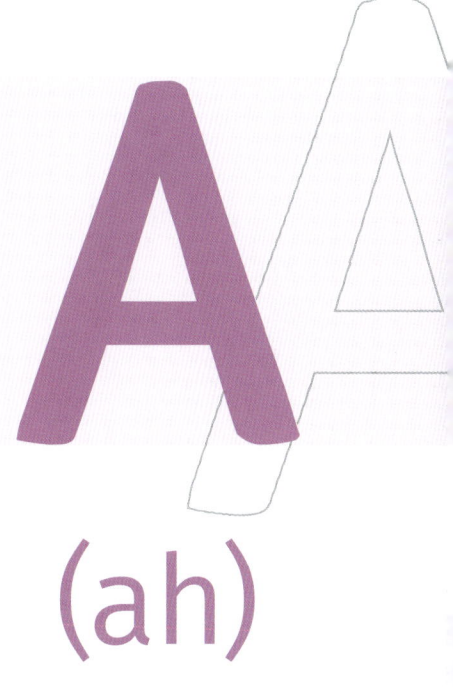

A (ah)

Opening

- ☼ Strengthens the upright stance
- ☼ Counteracts posture asymmetries
- ☼ Balances the inner and outer
- ☼ Harmonises inbreath and outbreath
- ☼ Balances building-up and breaking-down processes in the body
- ☼ Helps regulate sleep

Soul mood   Receiving, wonder, devotion

Vowel Exercises

Arm movement

- ☼ Speak or intone the sound three times
- ☼ Sense the open angle in your arm muscles
- ☼ Open yourself to the world, receptive to wonder

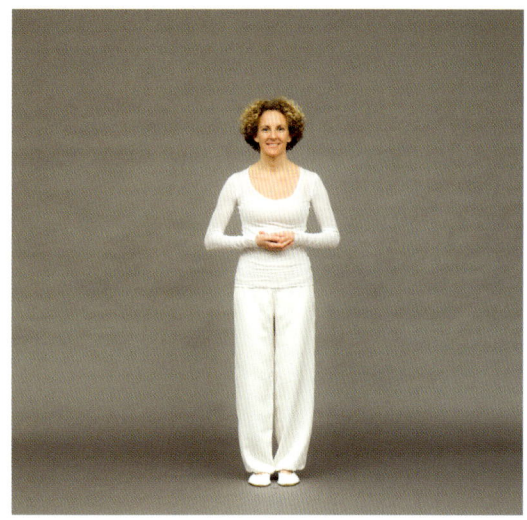

1 This is your basic starting position to begin any arm movement. Stand upright. Feel a connection to the earth with your feet. Keep your knees loose and breathe calmly. Cup your hands together, level with your diaphragm. Rest your gaze on the horizon. The movement impulse will emanate from your heart.

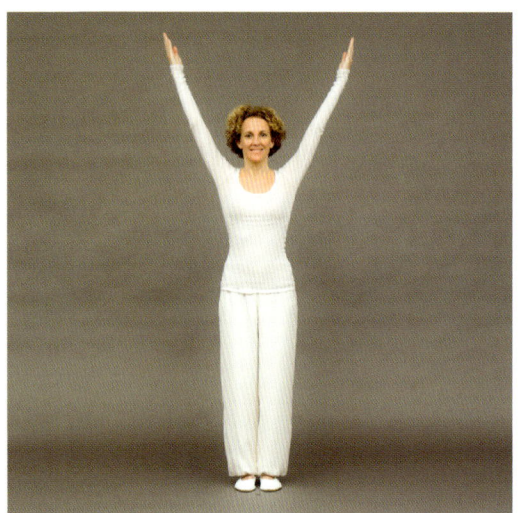

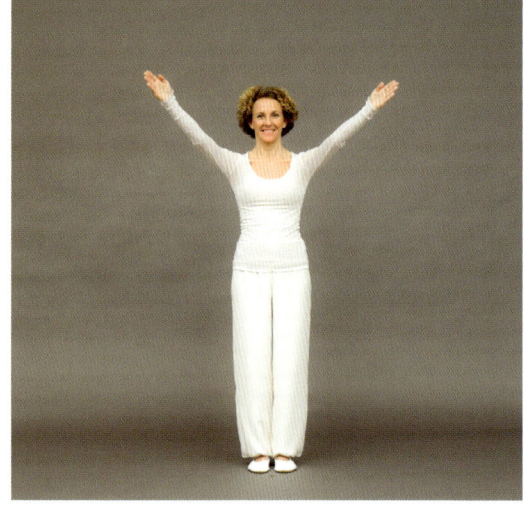

2 Raise your arms straight upwards and outwards. Sense the angle you are making. Release the arms and lead them back to the starting position.

3 Raise your arms again, but this time lower and slightly in front of you. Sense the angle as before. Then return to the starting position.

Vowel Exercises

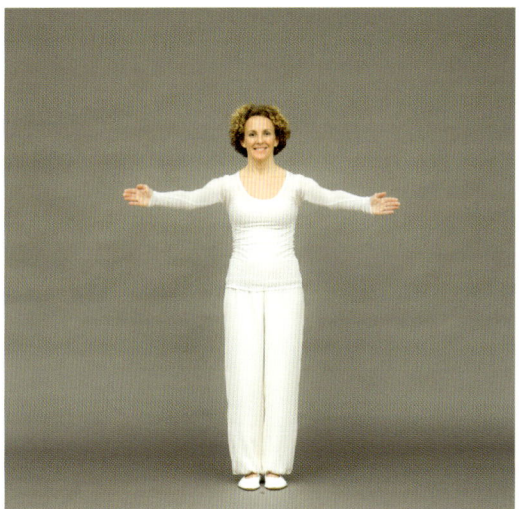

4 Form the same angle in the forward horizontal plane. Sense the angle in your arms. Return to the starting position.

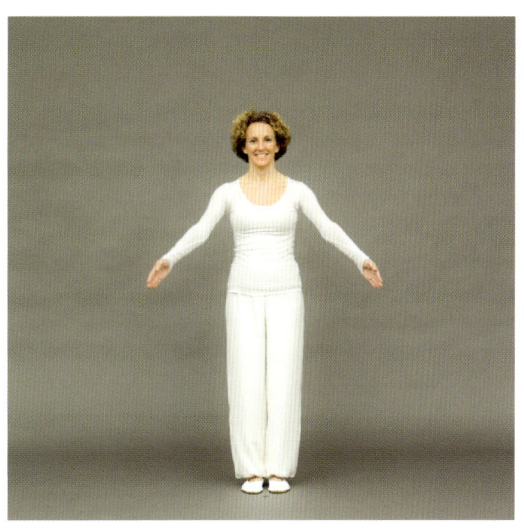

5 Form the same angle in the lower forward space. Sense the angle in your arms. Return to the starting position.

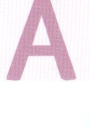

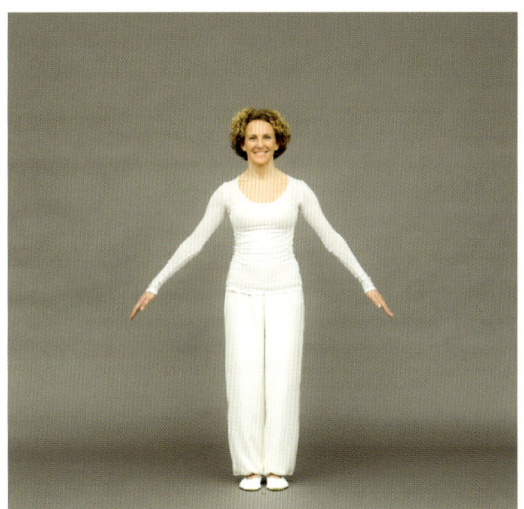

6 Now form the same angle directly downwards. Sense the angle in your arms. Then return to the starting position.

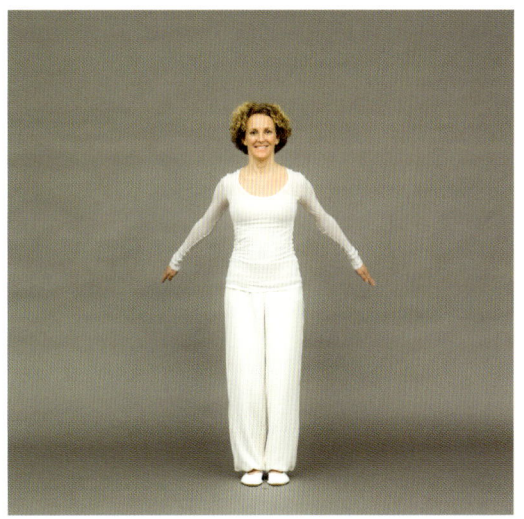

7 Finally, form the same angle downwards and slightly backwards. Sense the angle in your arms and return to the starting position.

Vowel Exercises

Swinging arms

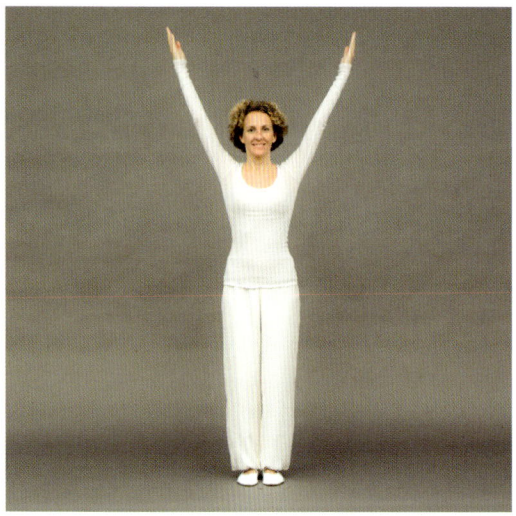

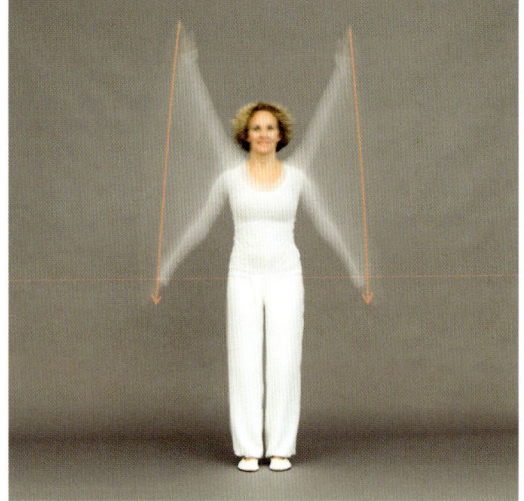

1 Raise your arms straight upwards and outwards...

2 ...and swing them down in front of you, moving into the space behind you. Hold here, feeling the angle in your arms, and then release. This can be repeated several times.

Vowel Exercises

Leg movement

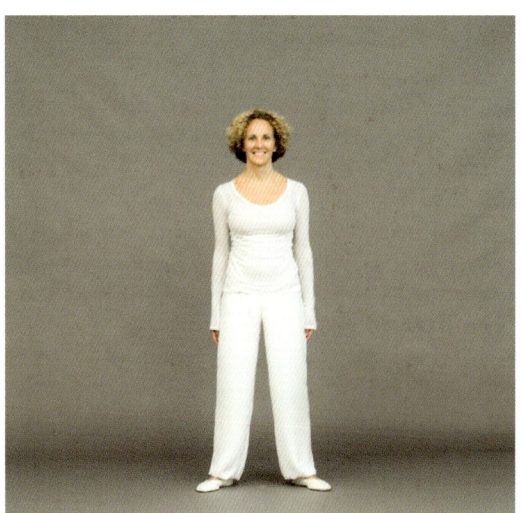

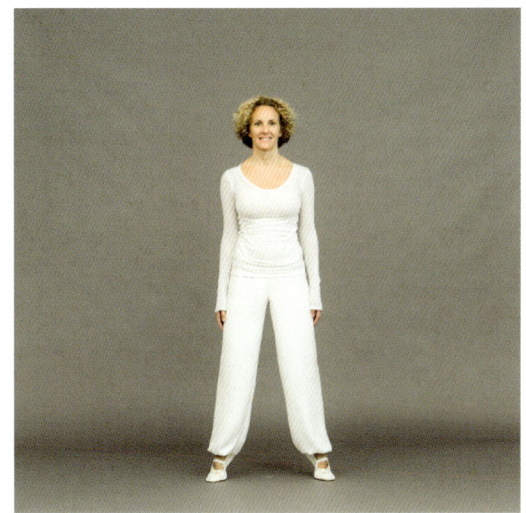

1 Form an A angle with your legs. Sense the angle you are making.

2 Rise up onto your toes, then lower yourself back down. Repeat as many times as you performed the arm movements. This can be done standing in place or after stepping forwards and backwards. After each step, bring your feet together again side by side.

Tip

☼ After doing the exercise, spend a moment listening to the vowel sound resonating within you.

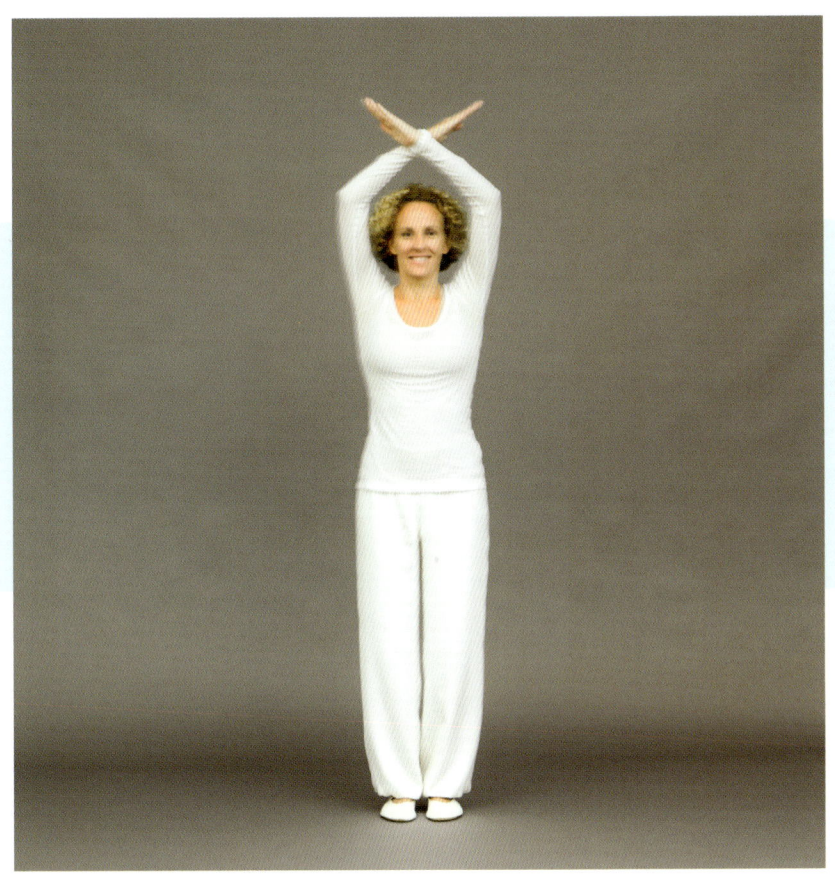 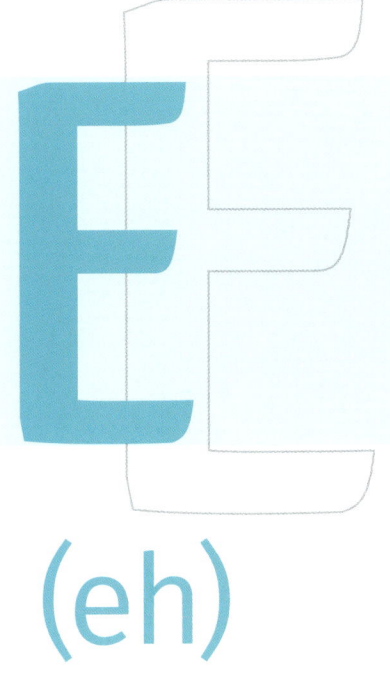

(eh)

Crossing

- ☼ Strengthens coordination and dexterity
- ☼ Counteracts postural asymmetries
- ☼ Helps generate warmth
- ☼ Centres, activates and grounds you
- ☼ Creates clear boundaries and strengthens defensive forces
- ☼ Strengthens our sense of self and self-perception
- ☼ Gives courage

Soul mood Self-assertion, wakefulness, reverence

Vowel Exercises

Arm movement I

- ☼ Speak or intone the sound three times
- ☼ Sense the crossing point of the E gesture
- ☼ Experience a centring impulse

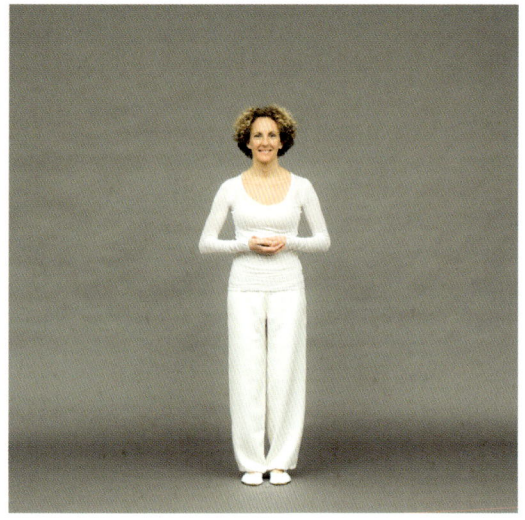

1 Stand upright. Feel a connection to the earth with your feet. Keep your knees loose and breathe calmly. Cup your hands together, level with your diaphragm. Rest your gaze on the horizon. The movement impulse will emanate from your heart.

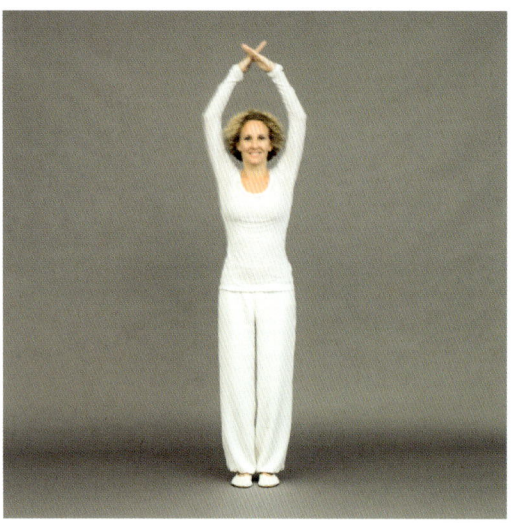

2 Keeping your fingers together, cross your hands over your head. Sense the point at which your knuckles meet. Release the arms and return them to the starting position.

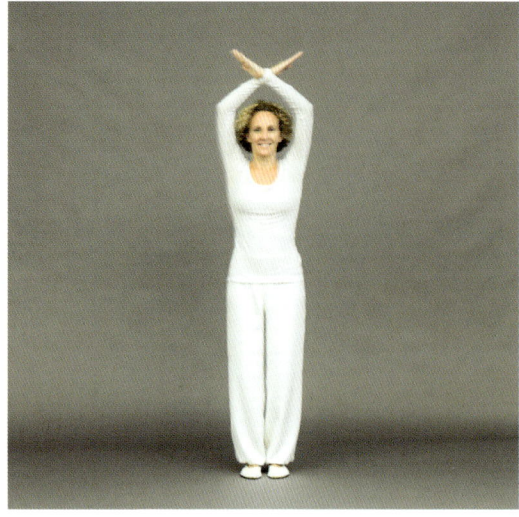

3 This time, cross your arms a little closer to your head, at the wrists. Sense the crossing point. Then return to the starting position.

Vowel Exercises

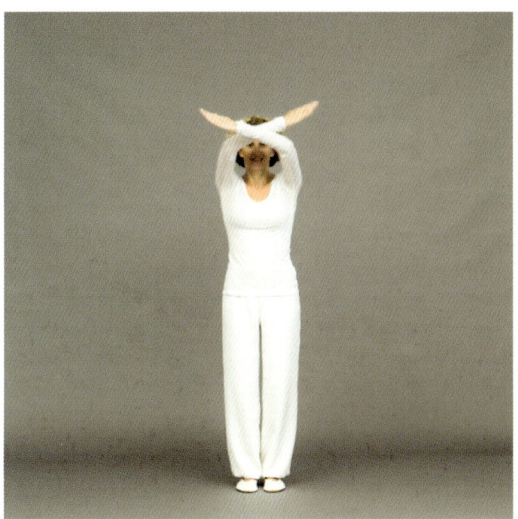

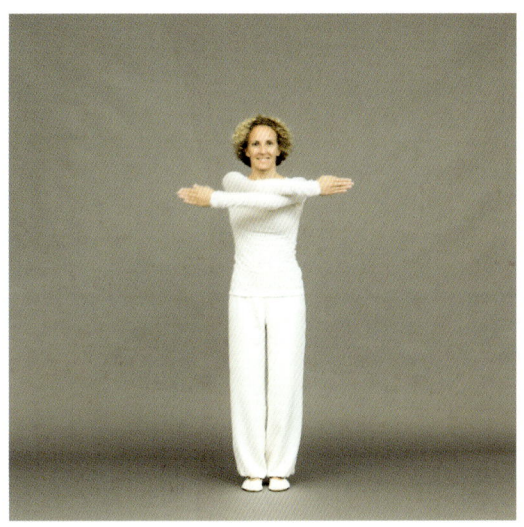

4 Cross your forearms in front of your face. Sense the crossing point. Return to the starting position.

5 Cross your elbows in front of your chest. Sense the crossing point. Return to the starting position.

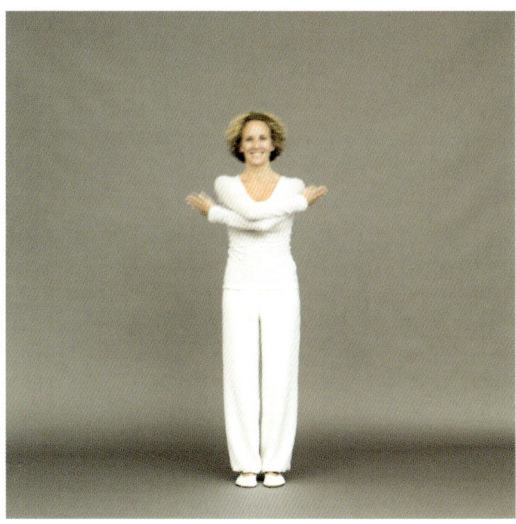

6 Lastly, cross your upper arms. Sense the crossing point and return to the starting position.

E

Vowel Exercises

Swinging arms I

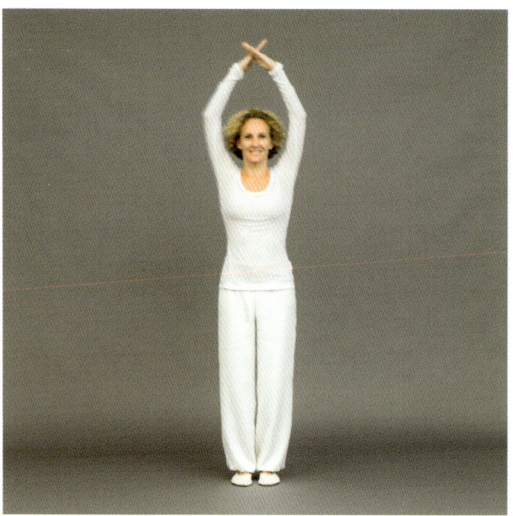

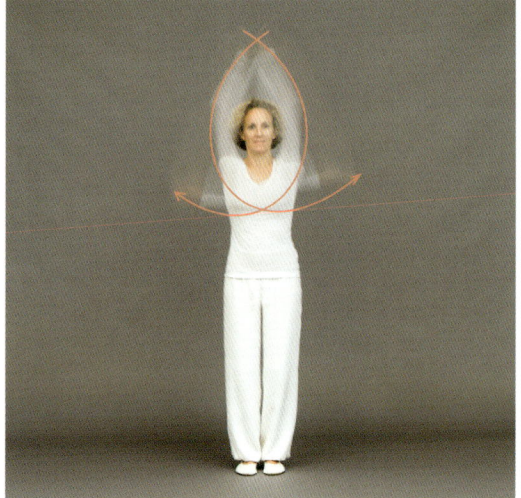

1 Begin as with your hands crossed above your head.

2 Swiftly bring your arms down and across your chest in one motion, crossing further and further along your arms as you move from high to low. Try to sense the meeting of your arms at every point. This can be repeated several times.

Vowel Exercises

Leg movement I

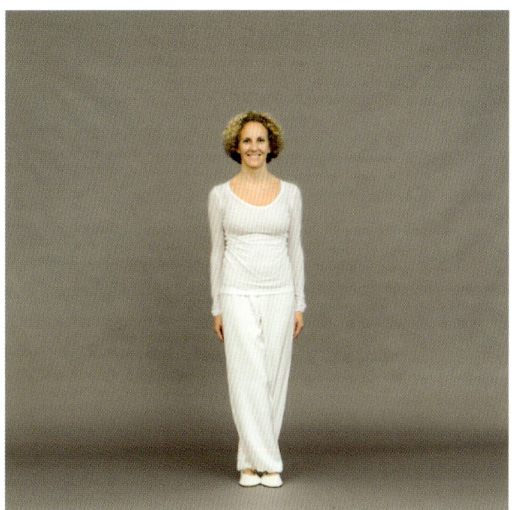

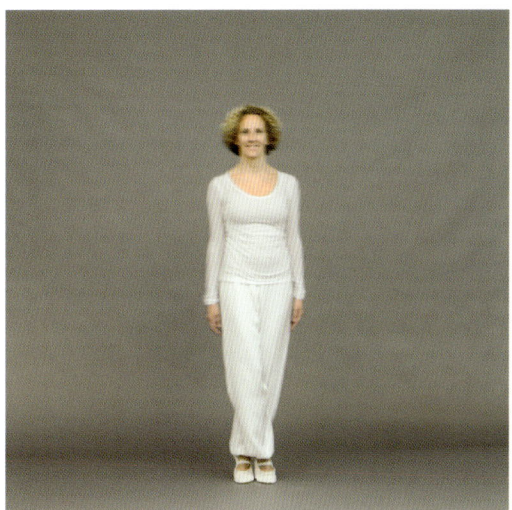

1 Cross your right leg over your left. Sense the point at which they meet.

2 Rise up on your toes, then lower yourself back down. Now cross the left leg over the right and repeat. Do this the same number of times as you did the arm movements, either standing in place or with a forward or backward step with both feet in between each motion.

Tip

✿ After doing the exercise, spend a moment listening to the vowel sound resonating within you.

Vowel Exercises

Arm movement II

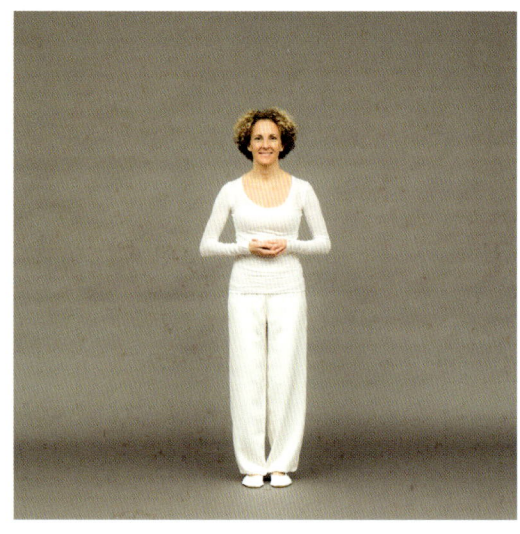

1   Starting position: Begin as you did in the 'E' arm movement 1 on page 24.

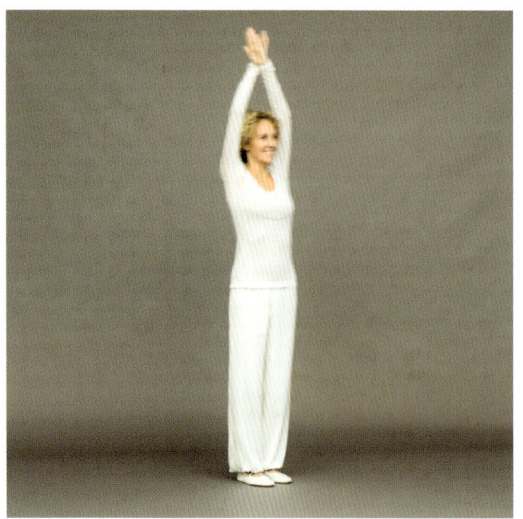

2   This variation keeps your arms crossed at your wrists for each gesture. First cross them above your head, sensing the point at which they meet. Release your arms and return to the starting position.

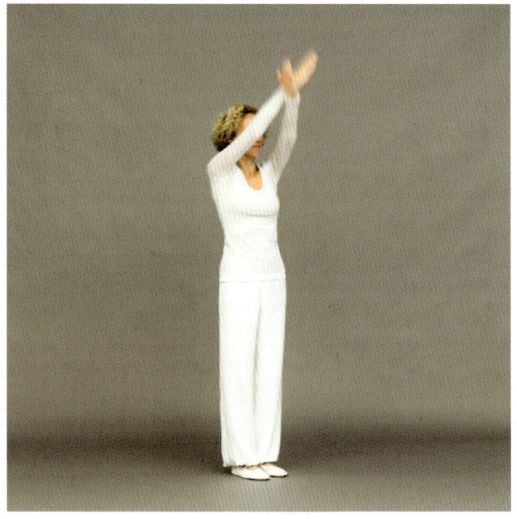

3   Now cross your wrists in front of you, level with your forehead. Sense the crossing point. Return to the starting position.

Vowel Exercises

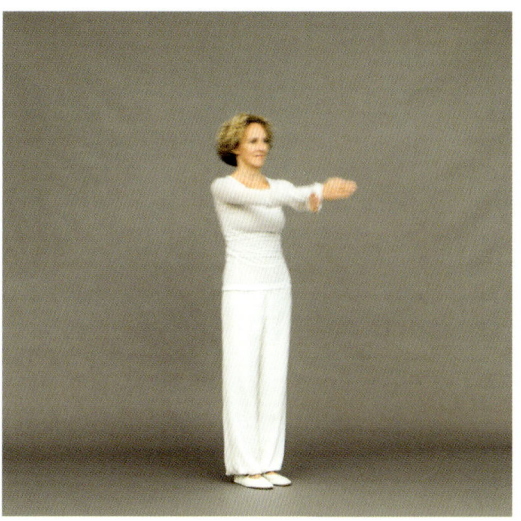 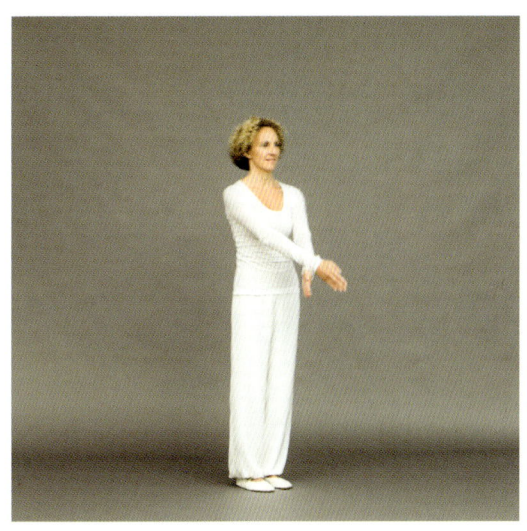

4 Cross your wrists horizontally in front of you, level with your heart. Sense the crossing point. Return to the starting position.

5 Now cross your wrists level with your abdomen. Sense the crossing point. Return to the starting position.

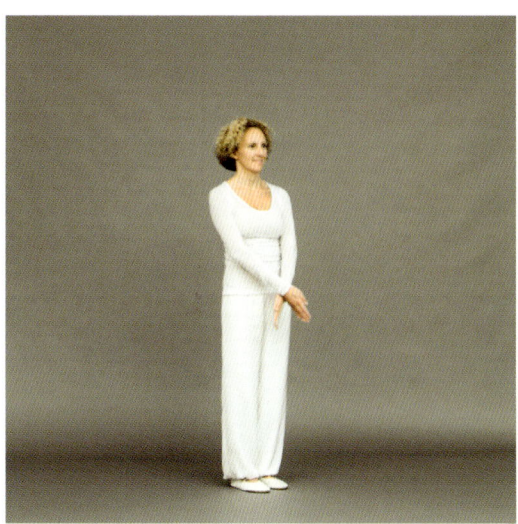

6 Finally, cross your wrists as far down as they will comfortably go. Sense the crossing point and return to the starting position.

E

Vowel Exercises

Swinging arms II

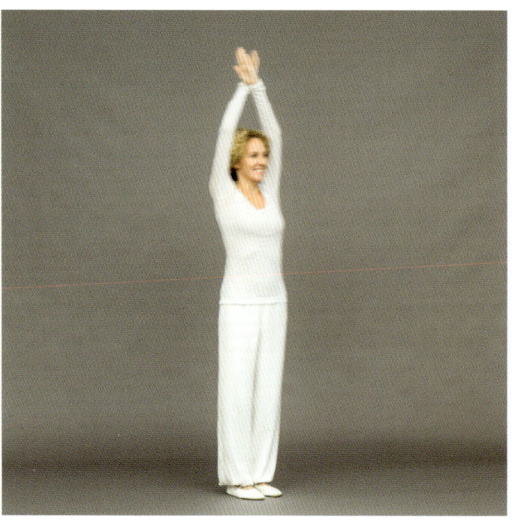 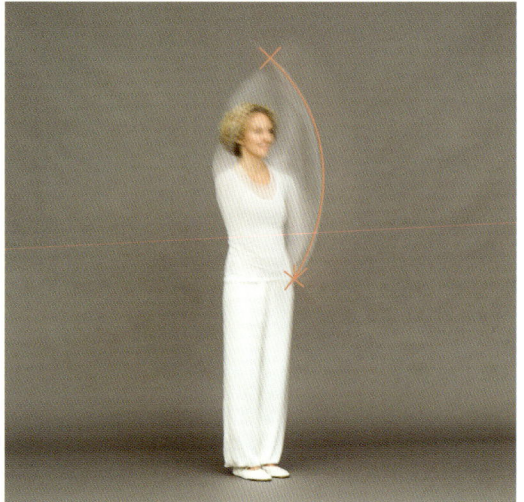

1 Begin with your wrists crossed above your head.

2 Now swing your arms down in an arc, keeping your wrists together. Sense the crossing point throughout the movement, and release at the bottom. This can be repeated several times.

Vowel Exercises

Leg movement II

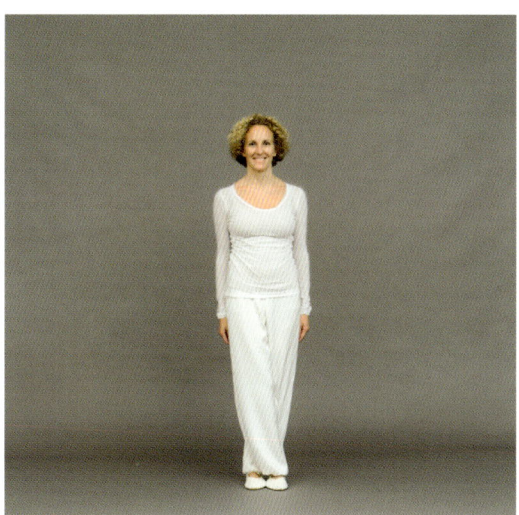

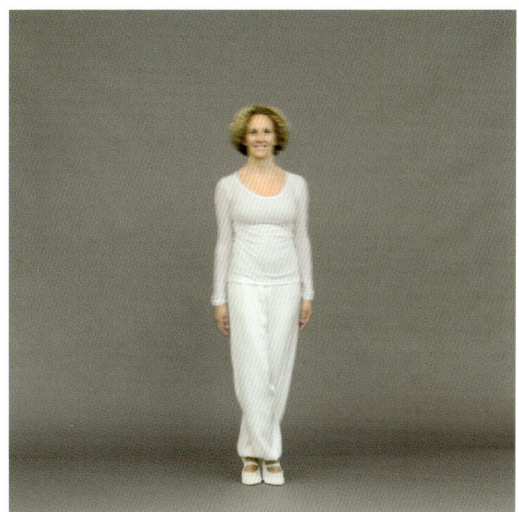

1 Cross your right leg over your left. Sense where they meet.

2 Rise up on your toes, then lower yourself back down. Now cross the left leg over the right and repeat. Keep alternating the movement the same number of times as you did with your arms. You can do this standing in place or with a full step (both feet) forwards or backwards between each crossing.

Tip

✷ Remember to listen to the vowel sound resonating within you.

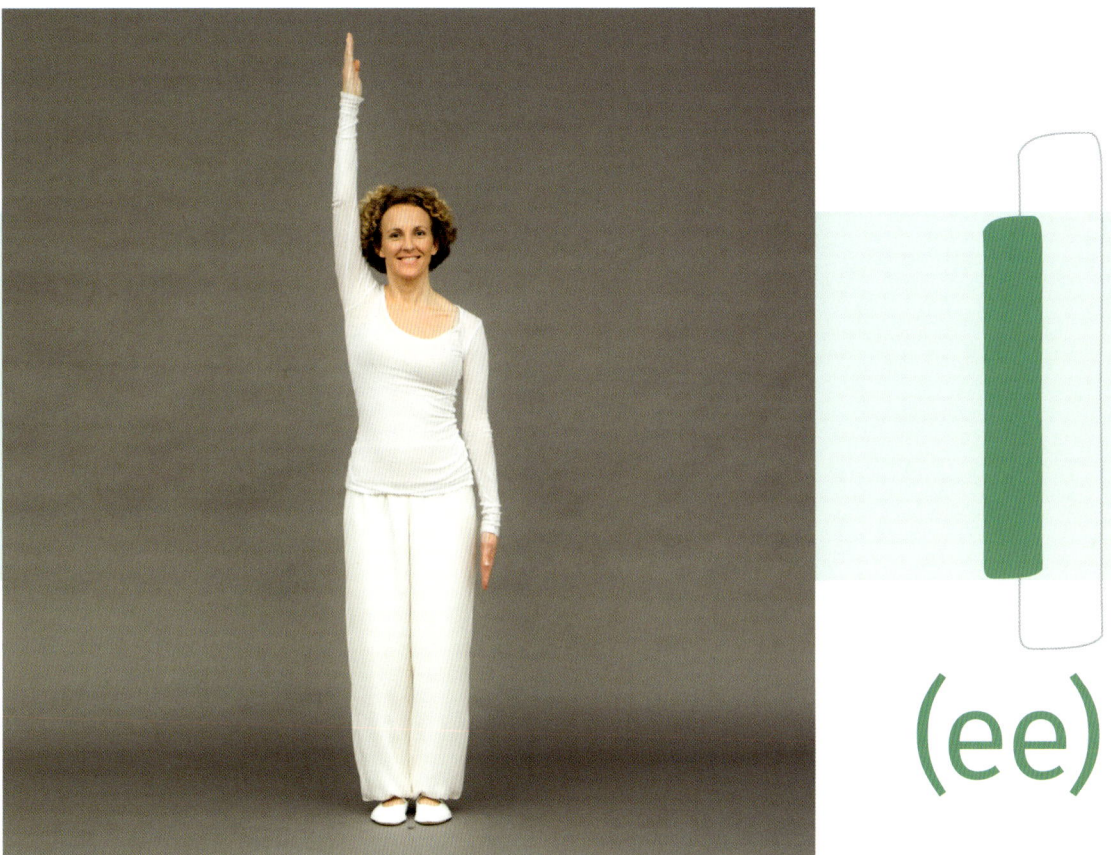

(ee)

Reaching out from the heart space

- ☼ Counteracts postural asymmetries and disorders; strengthens the upright back
- ☼ Supports a steady gait
- ☼ Improves balance
- ☼ Strengthens immune defence
- ☼ Improves psychological resilience
- ☼ Allows for inner mobility
- ☼ Helps the mind orientate between polarities and act with clear intention

Soul mood   Light-filled, radiant, balancing between tensions

Vowel Exercises

Arm movement

- ☼ First speak or intone the sound three times
- ☼ Sense a stretching in two opposite directions
- ☼ Perceive the lightening of the self
- ☼ Experience a radiant gesture

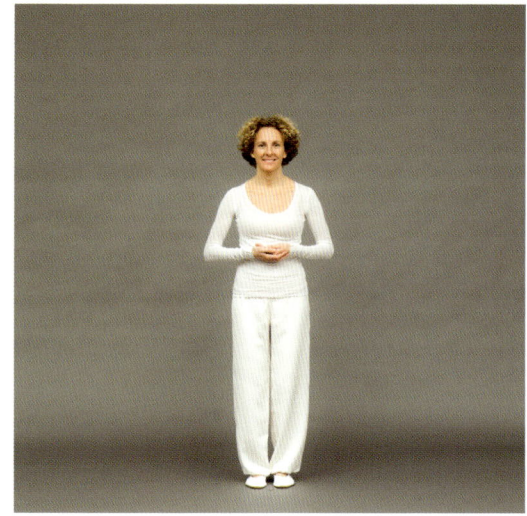

1 Stand upright. Feel a connection to the earth with your feet. Keep your knees loose and breathe calmly. Cup your hands together, level with your diaphragm. Rest your gaze on the horizon. The movement impulse will emanate from your heart.

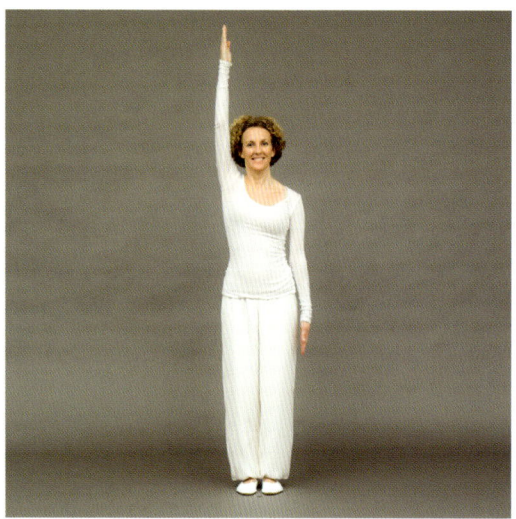

2 Extend the right arm upwards and the left arm downwards. Sense the continuity of this stretch through the arms. Release the arms and return to the starting position.

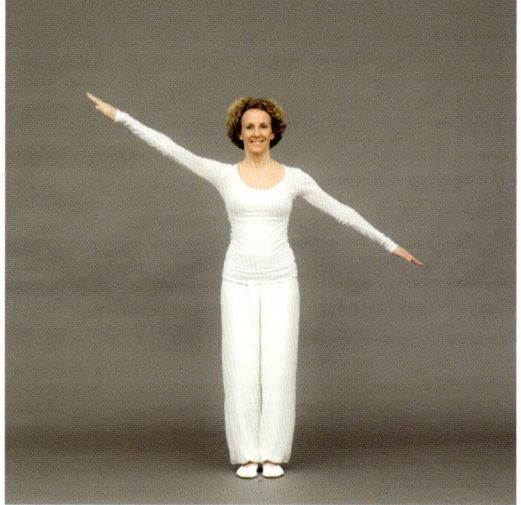

3 Extend the right arm diagonally upwards and the left diagonally downwards. Sense the continuity of the stretch. Return to the starting position.

Vowel Exercises

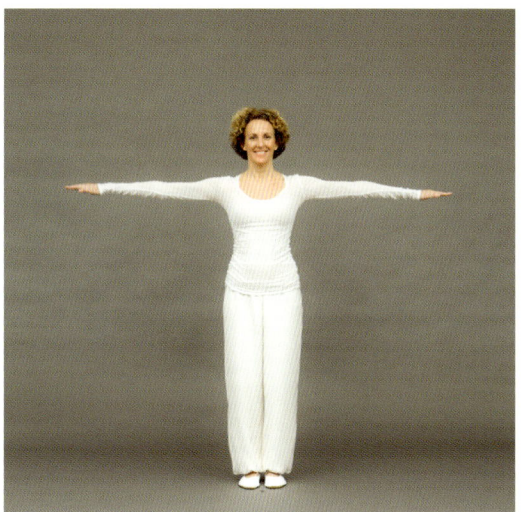

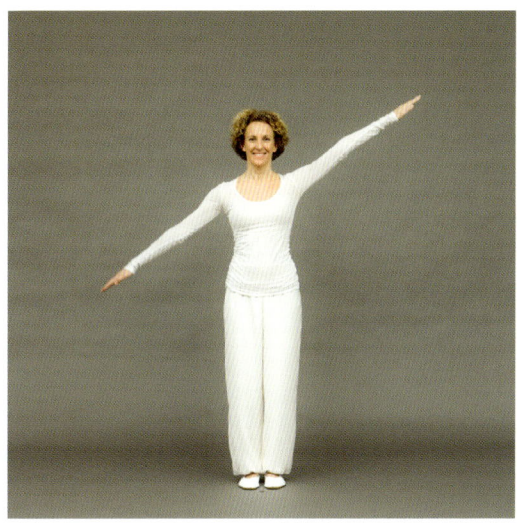

4   Extend both arms horizontally out to the sides. Sense the continuity of the stretch. Return to the starting position and rest.

5   Extend the right arm diagonally downwards and the left diagonally upwards. Sense the continuity of this stretching through the arms. Then return to the starting position.

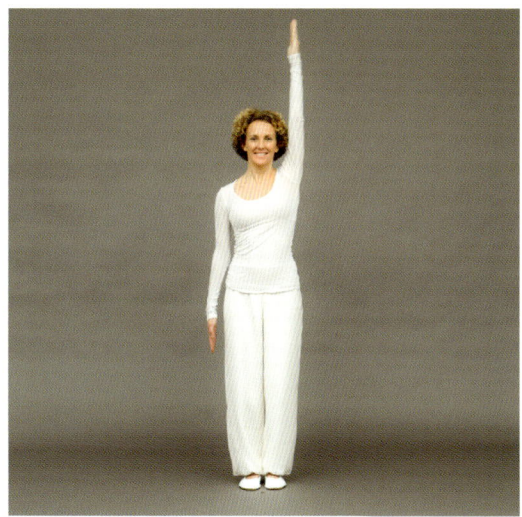

6   Extend the right arm downwards and the left upwards. Sense the continuity of this stretching through the arms. Then return to the starting position.

Tip

✿ You are free to extend this routine by adding stretches at intermediary diagonal angles.

Vowel Exercises

Swinging arms

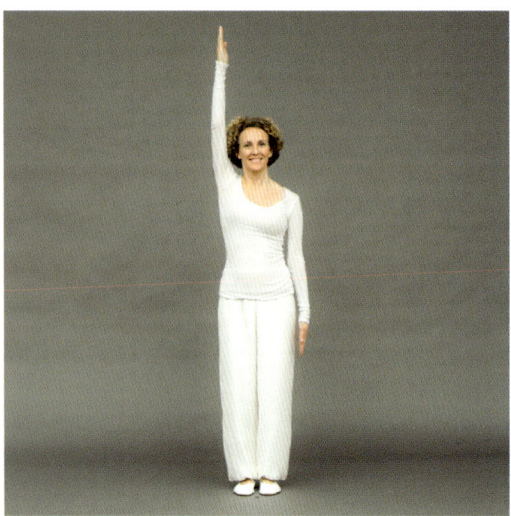 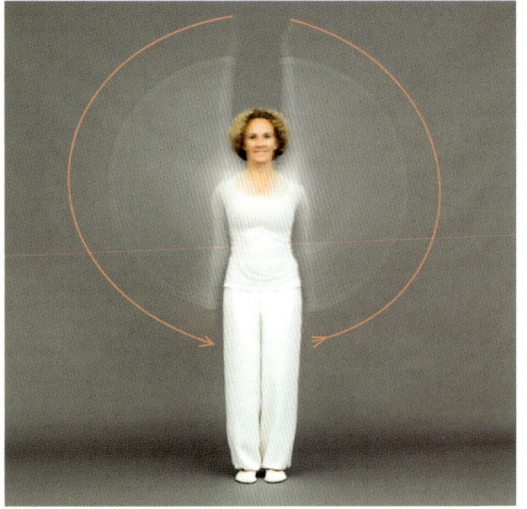

1 Extend the right arm upwards and the left downwards. Sense the continuity of this stretch through the arms.

2 At the same time, swing your right arm downwards and your left arm upwards, reaching out to the sides as you go. Repeat in the other direction, speeding up each time. End the swinging in your starting position. Sense any reverberation, and release.

Vowel Exercises

Leg movement I

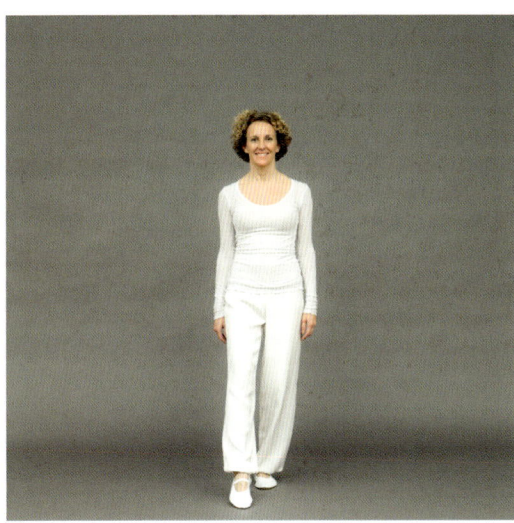

1 Alternately extend the right and the left leg forwards. You can do this standing in place or with a step forwards or backwards, bringing the feet together, in between each motion.

Tip

✿ Remember to spend a moment listening to the vowel sound resonating within you.

37

Vowel Exercises

Leg movement II

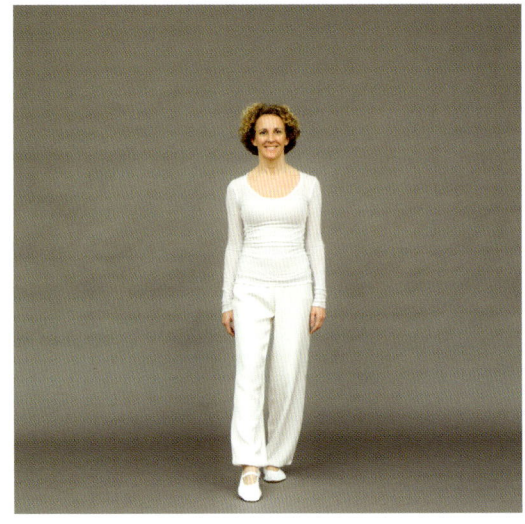

1 Extend your right leg forwards and sense the stretch. Release and return to a neutral standing position.

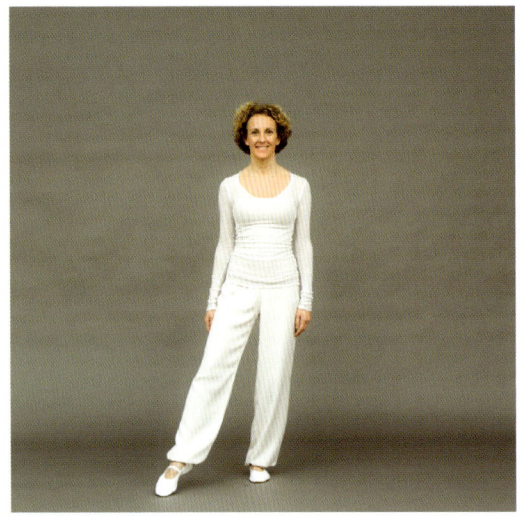

2 Extend your right leg forwards and to the side. Sense the stretch. Release and return to neutral.

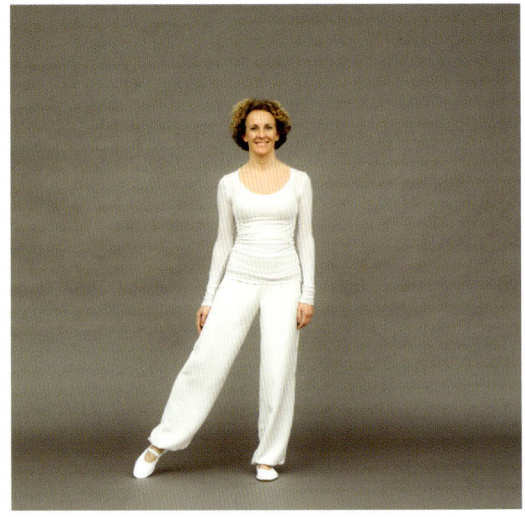

3 Extend your right leg sideways. Sense the stretch. Release and return to neutral.

Vowel Exercises

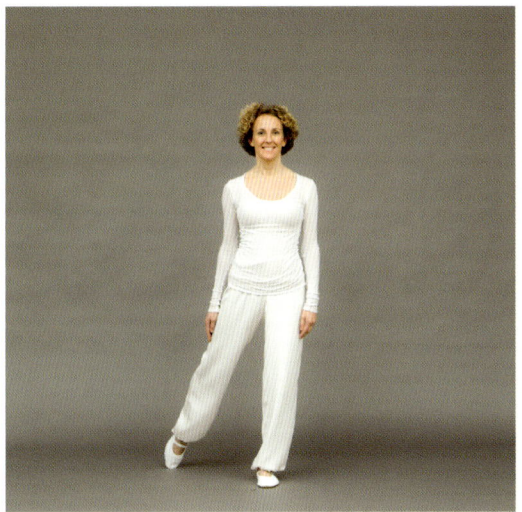

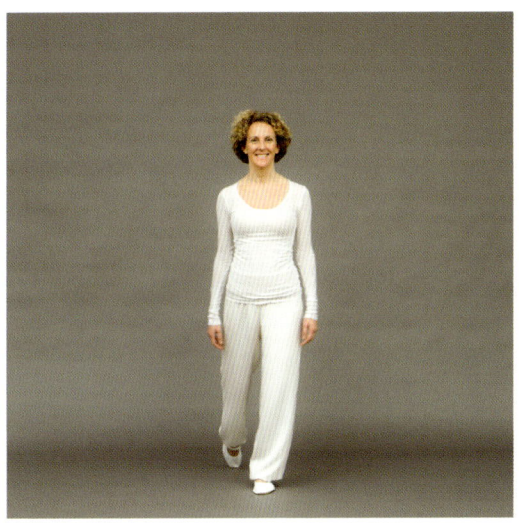

4 Extend your right leg backwards and to the side. Sense the stretch. Release and return to neutral.

5 Extend your right leg backwards. Sense the stretch. Release and return to the starting position. Now perform the whole sequence with your left leg.

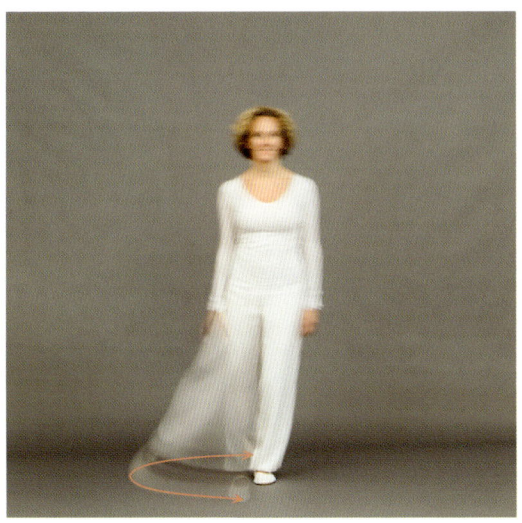

6 Imagine you are a sundial as you create one swift gesture from these smaller movements. Swing your extended right leg in a curve several times from front to back and forwards again, speeding up as you do so. End in front, release and return to neutral. Repeat the whole sequence with your left leg.

Tip

✺ Remember to listen to the vowel sound resonating within you.

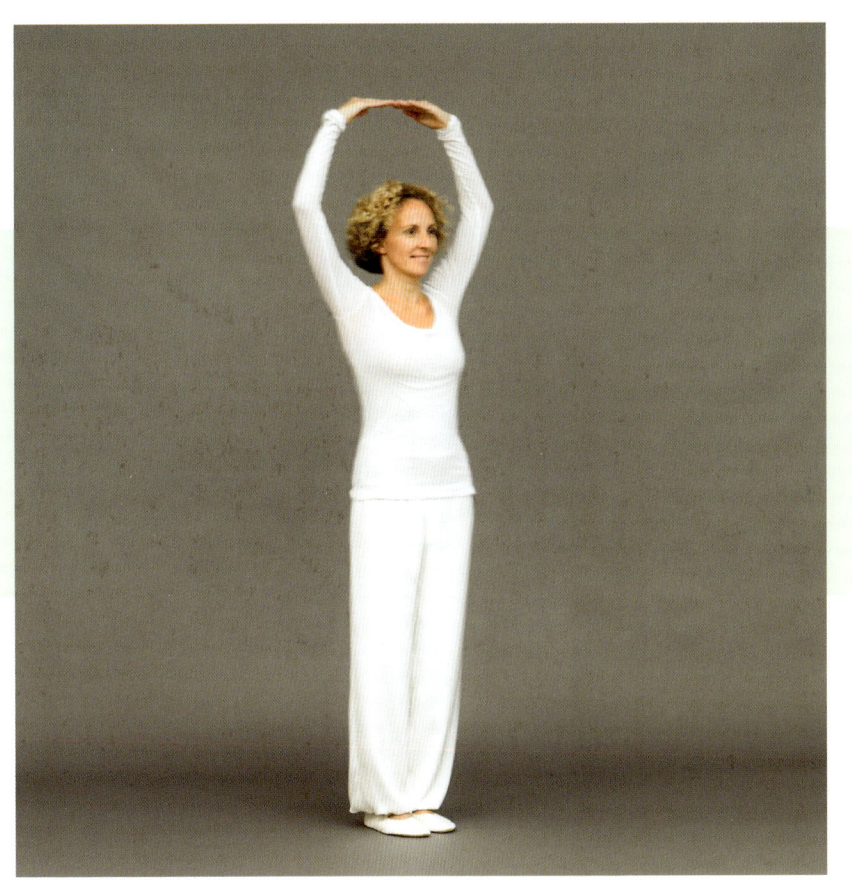

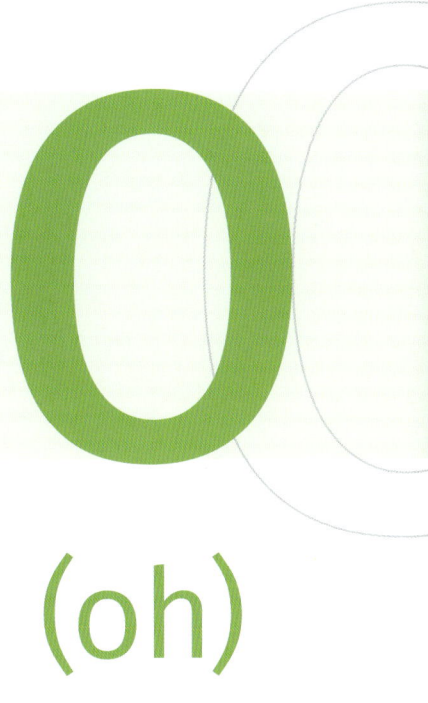

(oh)

Circular enclosing

- ☼ Harmonises the relationship between inner and outer self
- ☼ Creates a safe, peaceful interior space
- ☼ Nurtures inner calm and composure

Soul mood   Being at one with yourself, wellbeing, harmony

Vowel Exercises

Arm movement

- First speak or intone the sound three times
- Sense roundness in the muscles of your arms and legs
- Experience the encompassing nature of the gesture

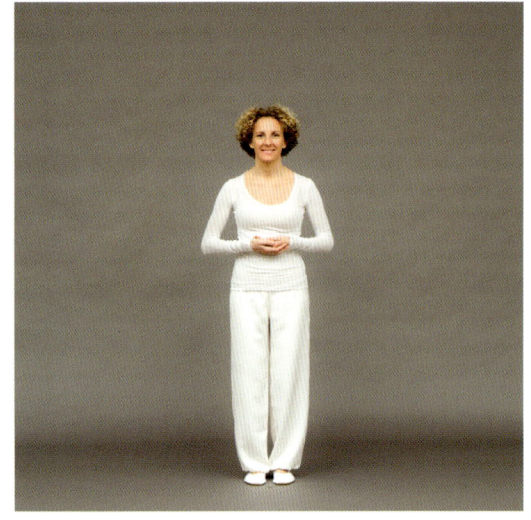

1 Stand upright. Feel a connection to the earth with your feet. Keep your knees loose and breathe calmly. Cup your hands together, level with your diaphragm. Rest your gaze on the horizon. The movement impulse will emanate from your heart.

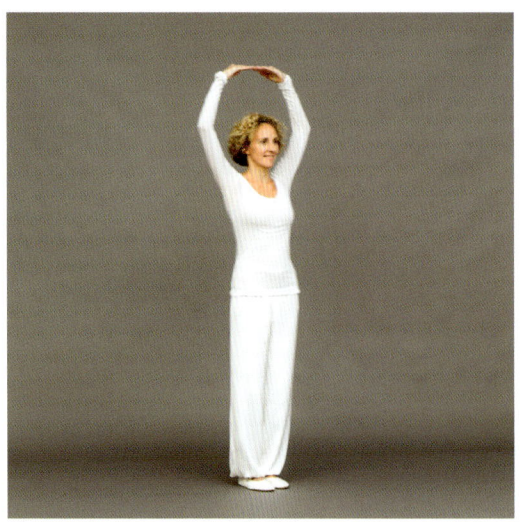

2 Form a circle with your arms above your head. Sense the roundness of your arms. Release and lead them back to the starting position.

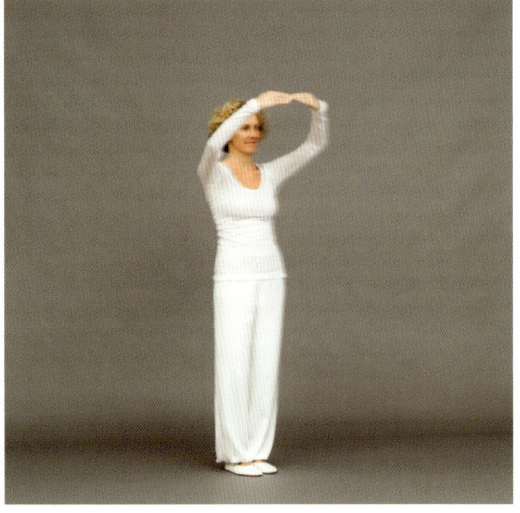

3 Form a slightly lower circle with the arms, so your hands are level with the top of your head. Sense the roundness of your arms. Return to the starting position.

Vowel Exercises

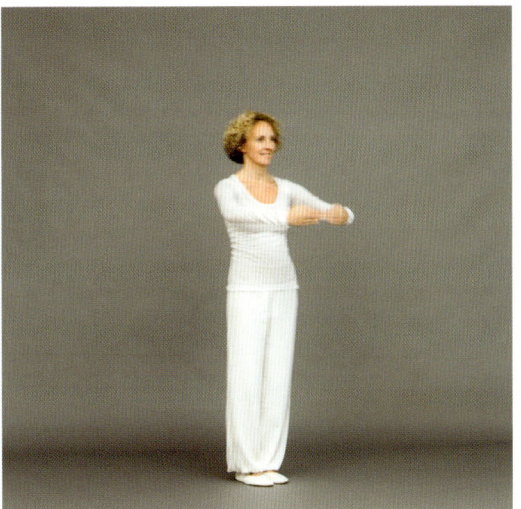

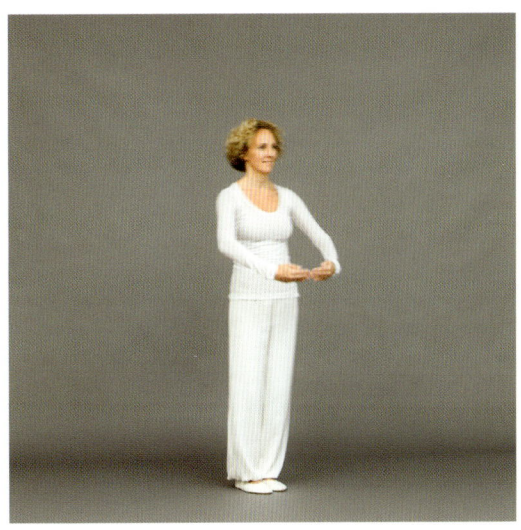

4   Form a circle with your arms in front of you, hands level with your heart. Sense the roundness of your arms. Return to the starting position.

5   Form a circle with your arms gently sloping downwards. Sense the roundness of your arms. Return to the starting position.

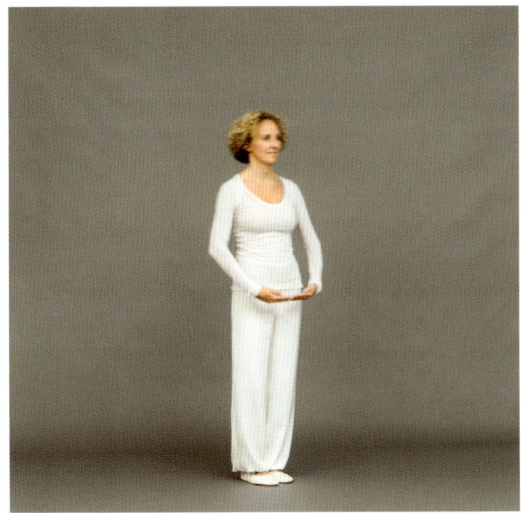

6   Lastly, form a circle with your arms completely downwards. Sense the roundness of the arms, release and return to the starting position.

Vowel Exercises

Swinging arms

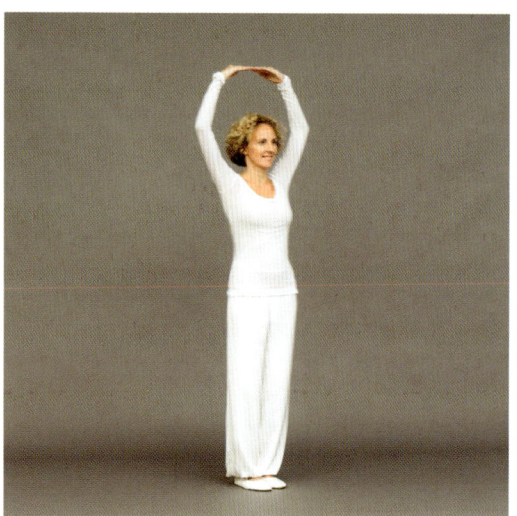 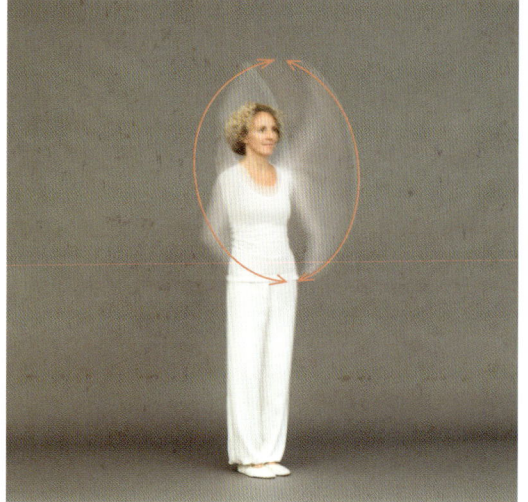

1 Form a circle with arms above your head. Sense the roundness of your arms as you prepare to swing the shape in front of you.

2 Swing your rounded arms downwards and upwards several times, speeding up as you go. End with the arms above your head, release and return to the basic starting position (see page 42).

Vowel Exercises

Leg movement

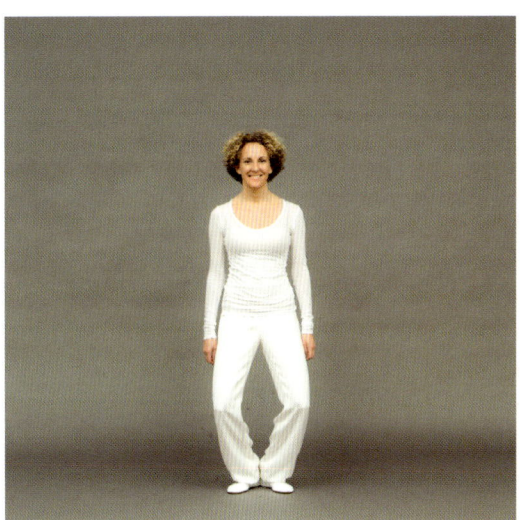 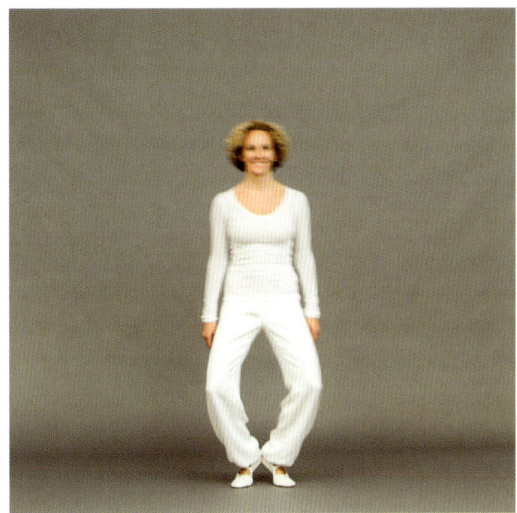

1 Turn your toes outwards while the heels touch. Bend your knees slightly and as you do so release the heels from the ground.

2 Rise onto your toes and down again as many times as you did the arm movements. Sense the roundness of the legs. You can do this standing in place or with a step in between each motion.

Tip

✿ Remember to spend a moment listening to the vowel sound resonating within you.

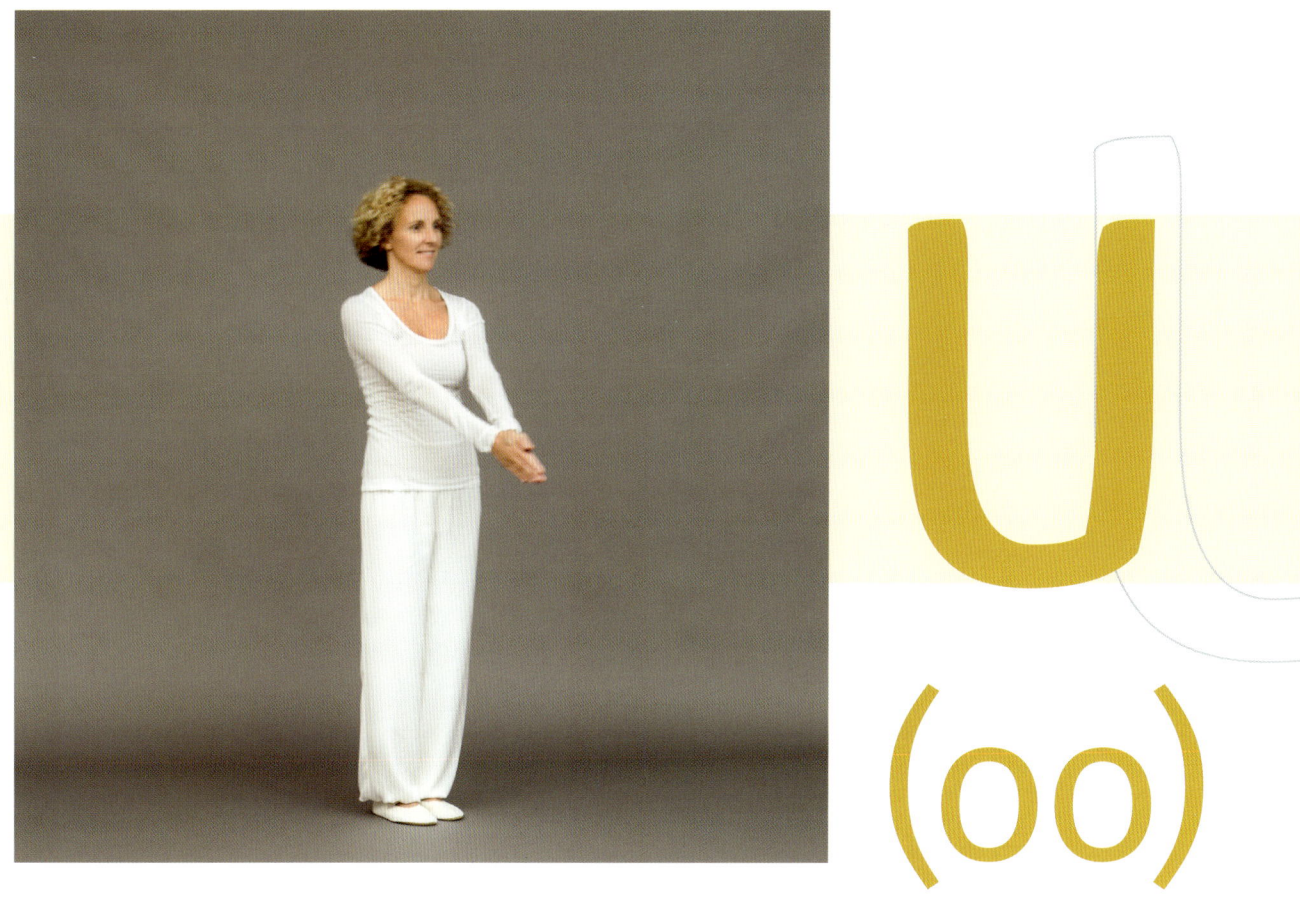

Bringing together

- Strengthens balance and stability
- Promotes inner and outer resilience
- Helps with posture
- Counteracts dizziness with clarity
- Promotes self-confidence

Soul mood Rootedness, self-reflection, equanimity

Vowel Exercises

Arm movement

- First speak or intone the sound three times
- Sense the parallel alignment of your arms or legs
- Experience a contracting gesture

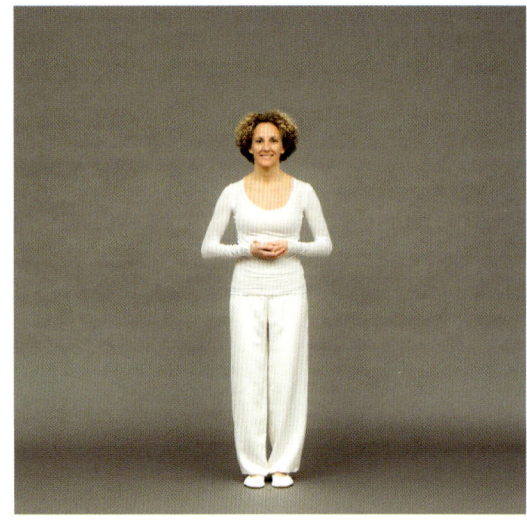

1 Stand upright. Feel a connection to the earth with your feet. Keep your knees loose and breathe calmly. Cup your hands together, level with your diaphragm. Rest your gaze on the horizon. The movement impulse will emanate from your heart.

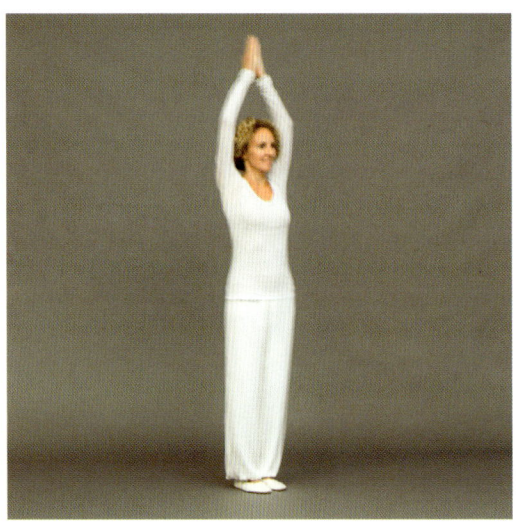

2 Bring your hands together high above your head. Sense the parallel quality of your arms. Release and return to the starting position.

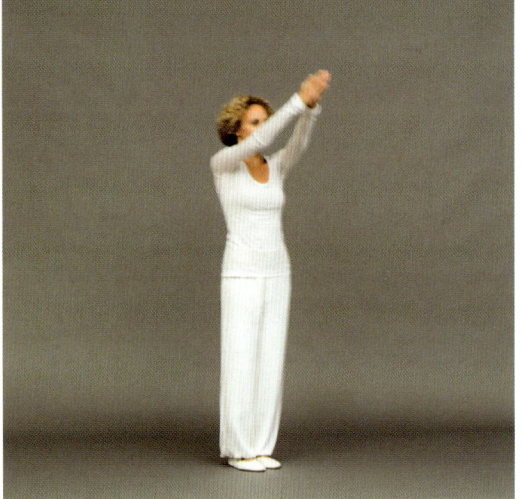

3 With palms touching, move your outstretched arms upwards and forwards. Sense the parallel quality of your arms. Return to the starting position.

Vowel Exercises

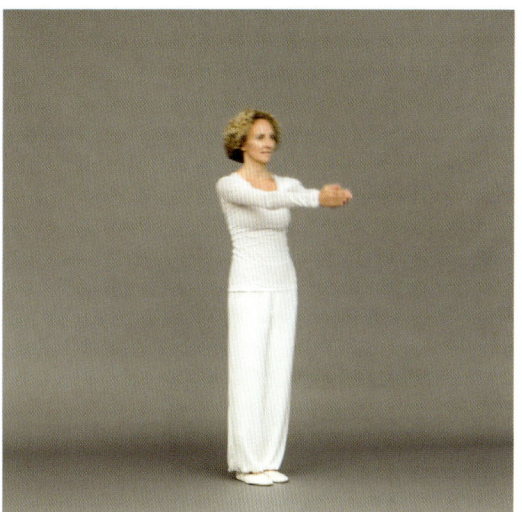 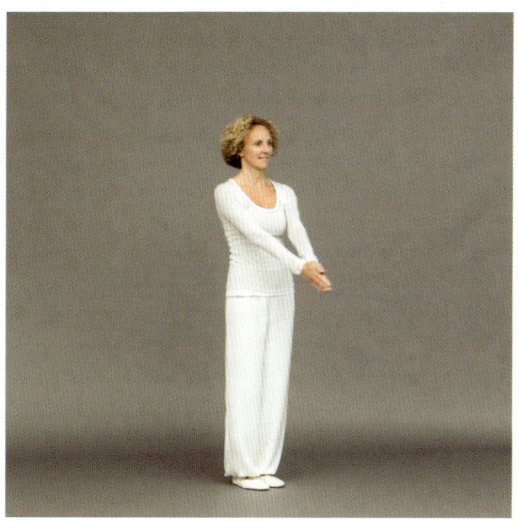

4 Now stretch your arms horizontally forwards, so your hands are level with your heart. Sense the parallel quality of the arms. Return to the starting position.

5 Stretch your outstretched arms forward and down, hands level with your hips. Sense the parallel quality of your arms. Return to the starting position.

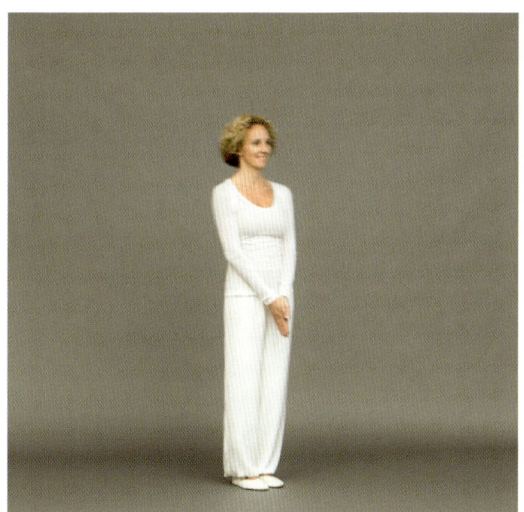

6 Lastly, stretch your arms straight downwards. Sense the parallel quality of your arms, release and return to the starting position.

U

Vowel Exercises

Swinging arms

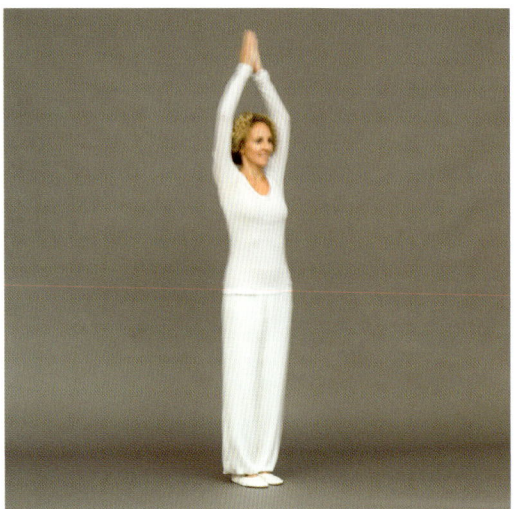

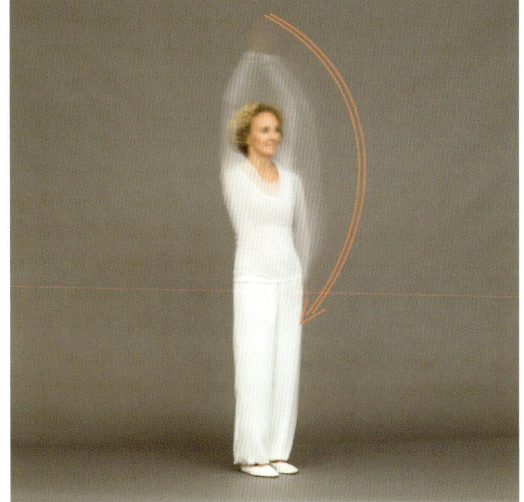

1 With palms touching, extend your arms high above your head. Prepare to sense the parallel quality in your arms as you sweep them down in front of you.

2 Swing your outstretched arms downwards and upwards several times, speeding up as you go. Finish with the arms back above your head. Release, return to the starting position on page 42 and rest.

Vowel Exercises

Leg movement I

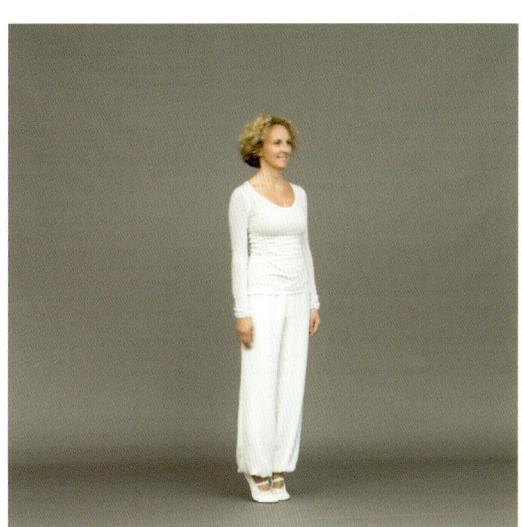

1 Stand with your legs together and arms by your sides. Sense the parallel quality in your legs as they support you. Rise onto your toes and down again as many times as you did the arm movements. You can do this standing in place or with a full step backwards or forwards between each movement.

Leg movement II

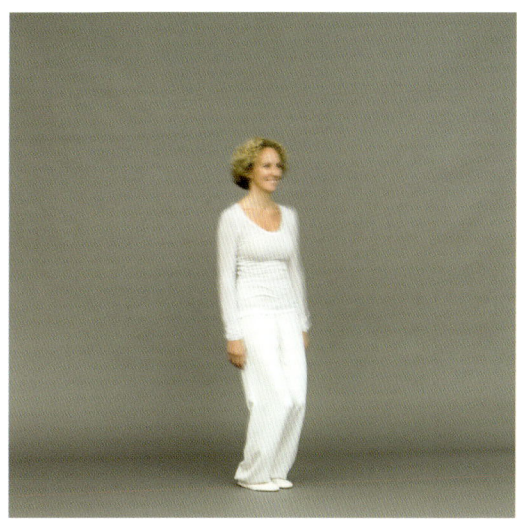

1 Stand with your legs together, sensing their parallel quality. Rise onto your toes and down again, then gently bend your knees and extend them again. You can repeat this on the spot or with steps as before.

U

Tip

✿ Remember to listen to the vowel sound resonating within you.

Vowel Exercises

Vowels at a Glance

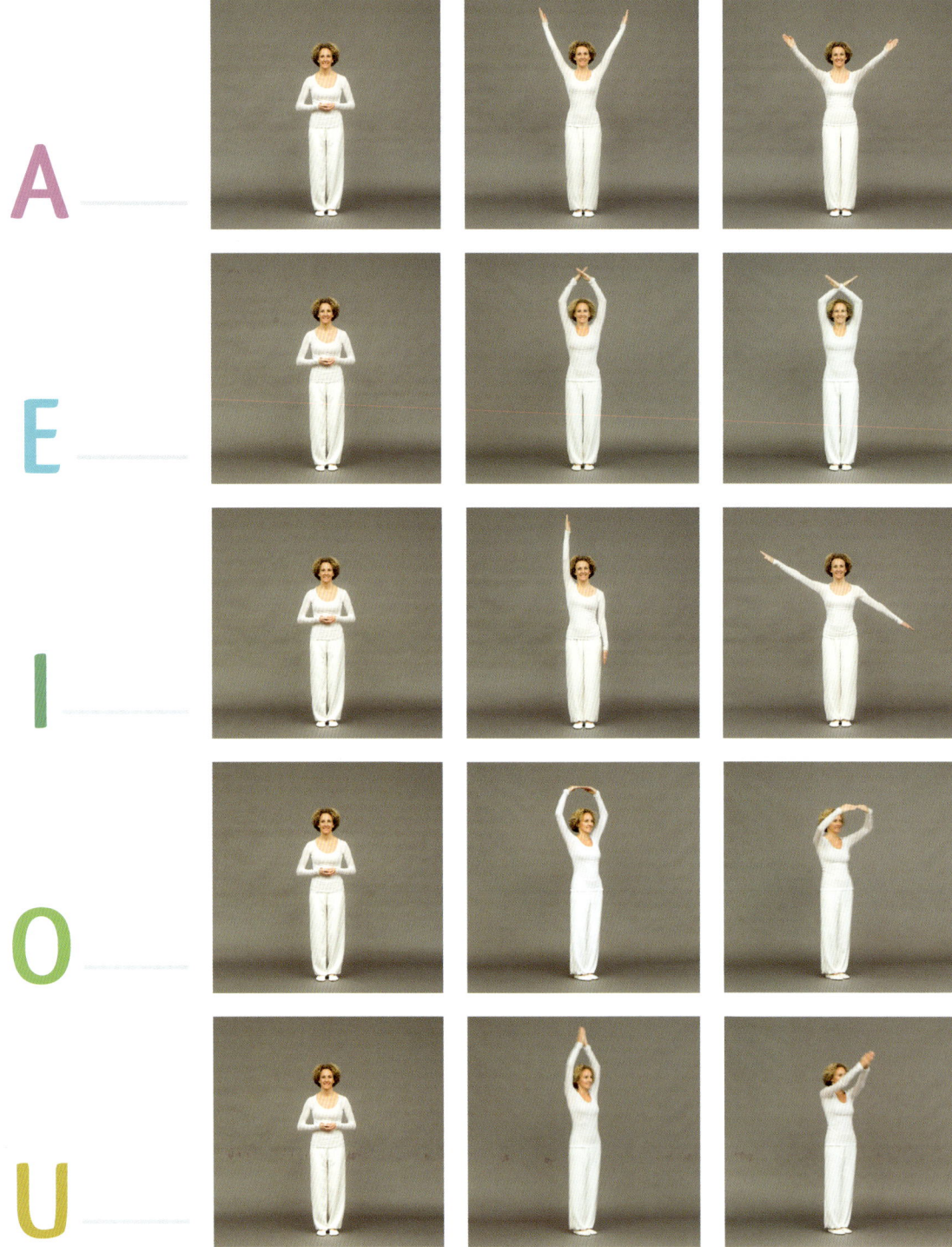

A

E

I

O

U

Vowel Exercises

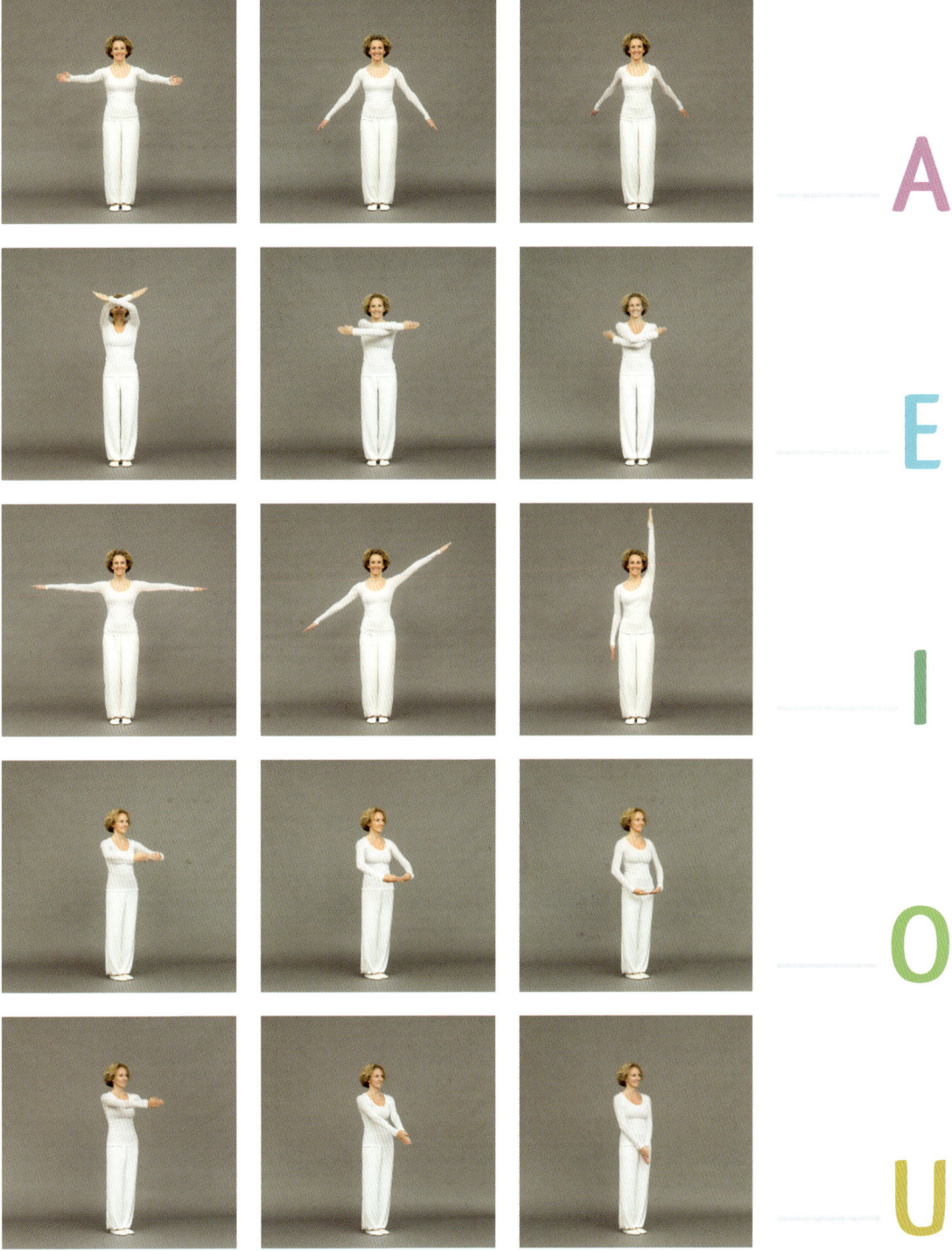

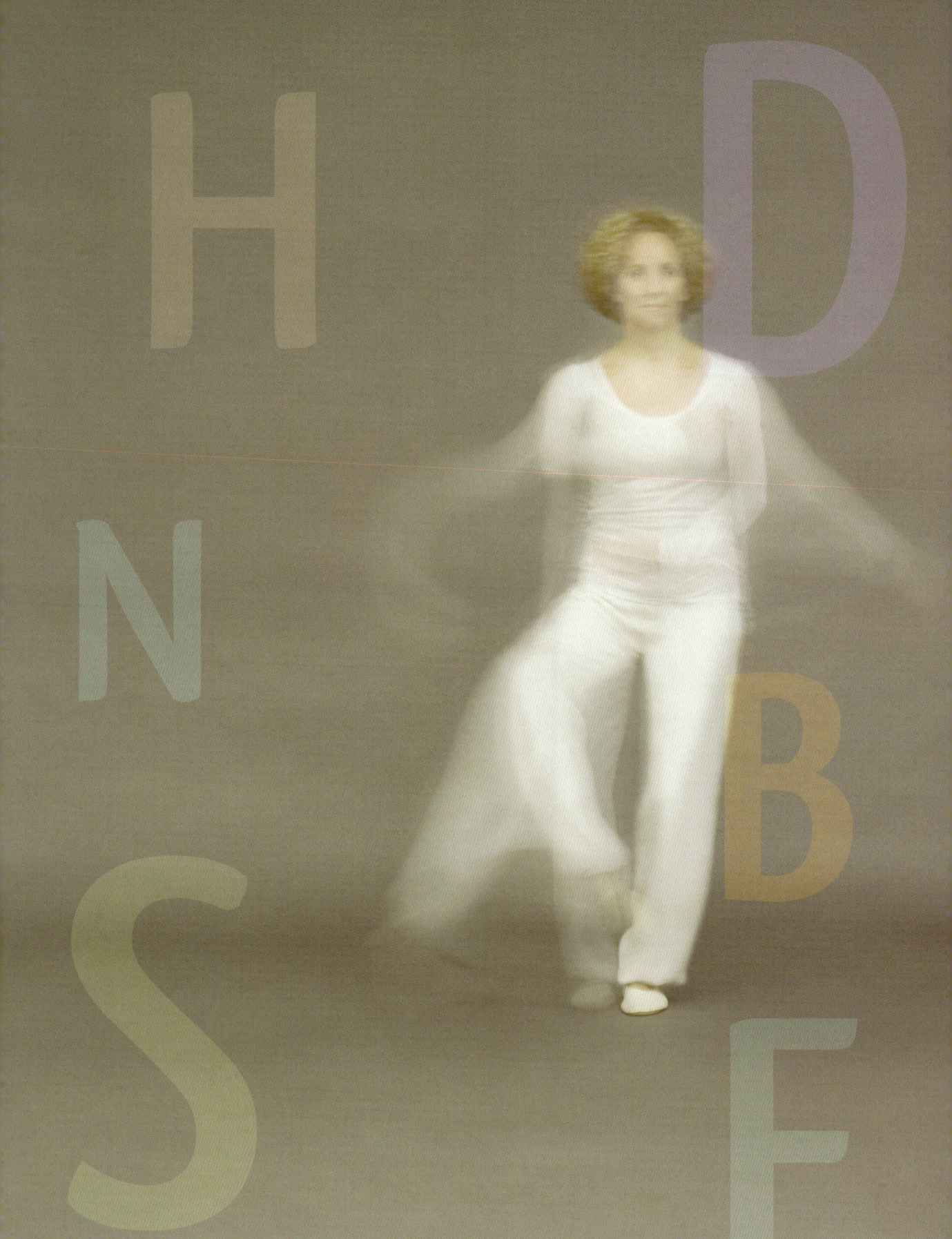

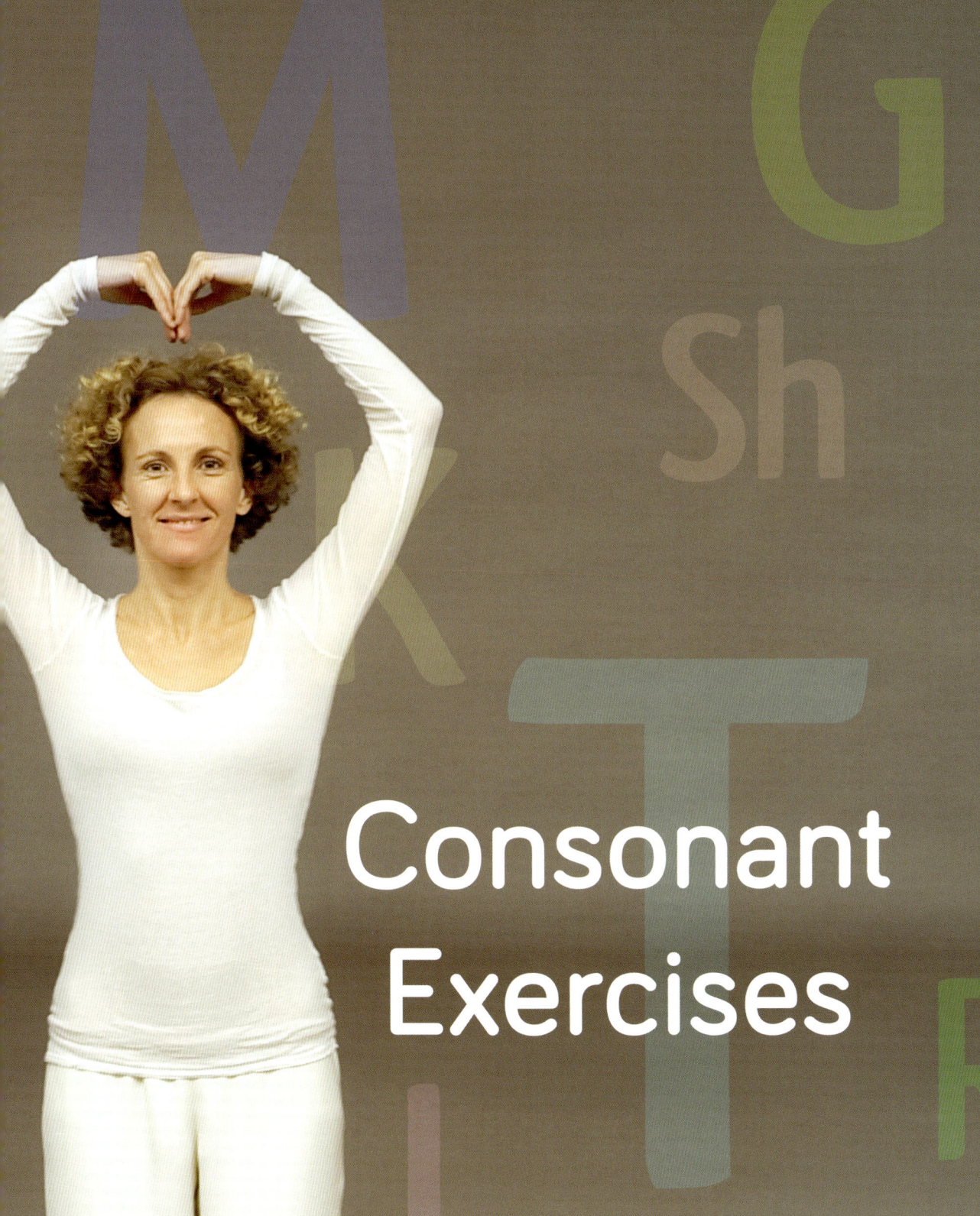

Consonant Exercises

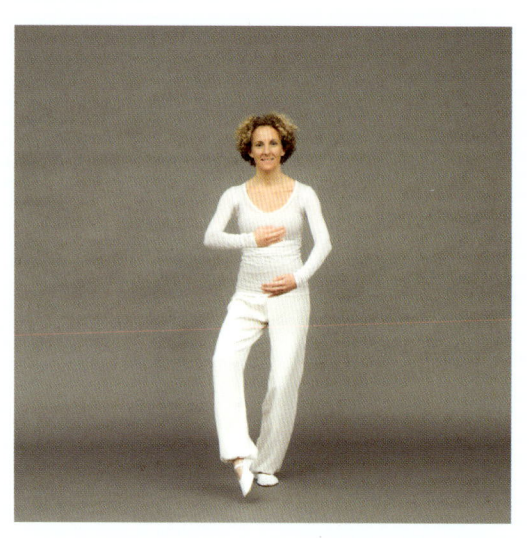
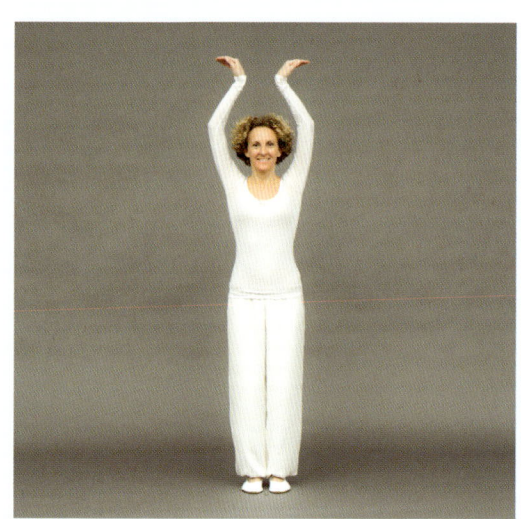
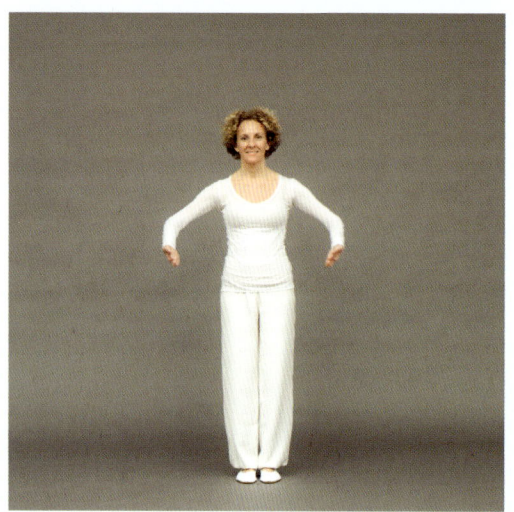
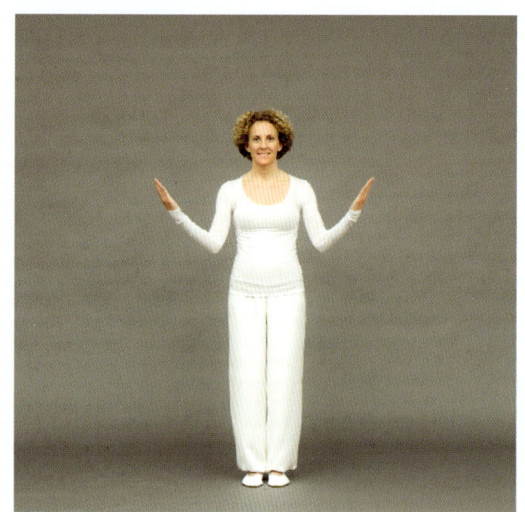

Getting started

Consonant exercises involve combining arm and leg movements simultaneously. We can add to our soul's experience of these by holding images of nature in our mind's eye while we do them.

Inner pictures

Everyone can recall a vivid memory of a sensory experience they once had in nature: a swift rushing stream; the salt-scented wind and surging waves of the seashore; a heavy mist rising in autumn; or the cracking and splintering of a branch breaking from a tree. Such experiences lie deep within us and are always within reach.

When we work with consonant sounds, we invoke these memories while we echo their living, dynamic sound in nature. Thus 'Sh' can express the rushing of water, 'F' the whistling of the wind, 'H' the melting of mist, and 'K' the hard crack of wood.

We can add to this by picturing ourselves in the scene, for example when we utter 'Sh', we imagine: 'I am standing in the surf, waves are breaking in front of me and rolling towards me, and I feel the salt spray in my face'.

As we move the sound, we can try to interact with the picture: 'Just as the air mingles with the breaking wave, I enter into the water and lead it in circling, spiral movements with my arms, from below upwards, where it becomes ever lighter and airier and finally dissolves'.

These exercises have their best effect when we are able to penetrate into the essence or archetype of a speech sound and its mode of action in such a way. The more vividly we can learn to experience it and shape it through gesture, the easier it is to recall again next time, allowing us more space to enjoy the experience.

Tips

- Each memory picture is unique to you, and yours to shape.
- Remember, the therapeutic effect takes place in the pause afterwards. Allow the consonant to carry on working in you.

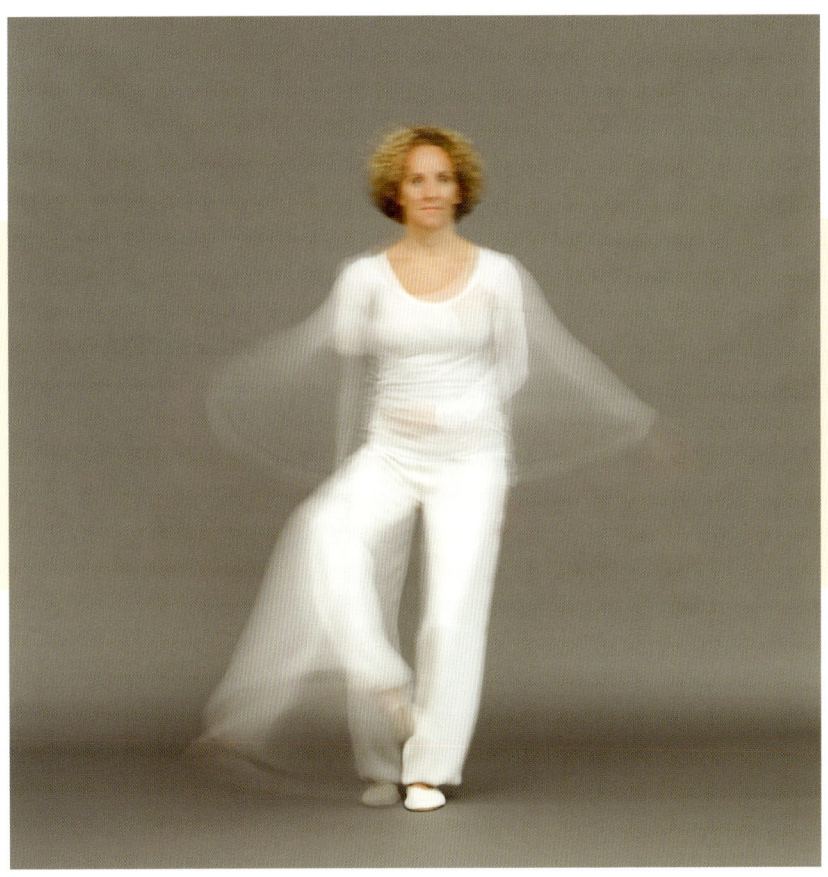 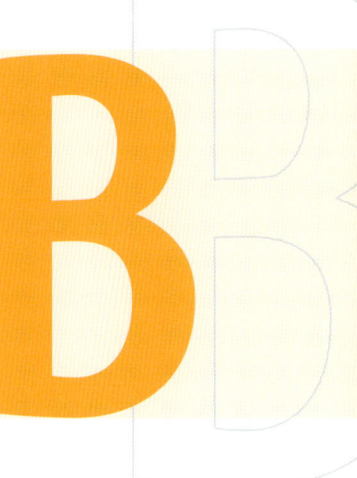

Enveloping and protecting

- ✺ Encourages warmth, calm, safety
- ✺ Creates and protects interior space
- ✺ Supports organ growth
- ✺ Protects a sense of self
- ✺ Has a qualitative affinity with P

Inner picture   Imagine placing a warm coat around you. Bring your arms in to hug your chest and protect your inner space. Repeat this gesture to further consolidate this protective space.

Arm movement

Tip

☼ The movement of the arms creates a protective form around your body, which encloses your inner space.

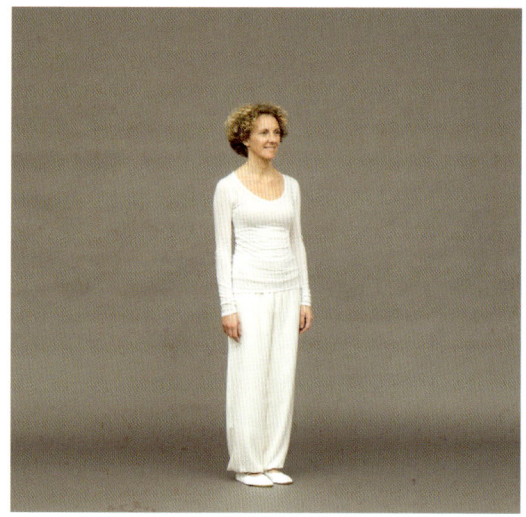

1 Stand upright. Feel a connection to the earth with your feet. Keep your knees loose and breathe calmly. Place your arms by your sides. Rest your gaze on the horizon. The movement impulse will emanate from your shoulder blades.

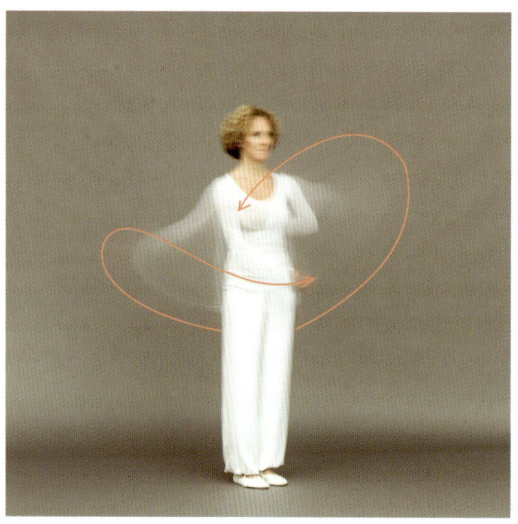

2 Move your arms in a sweeping, enclosing gesture in front of your upper body so that one arm comes to rest above the other.

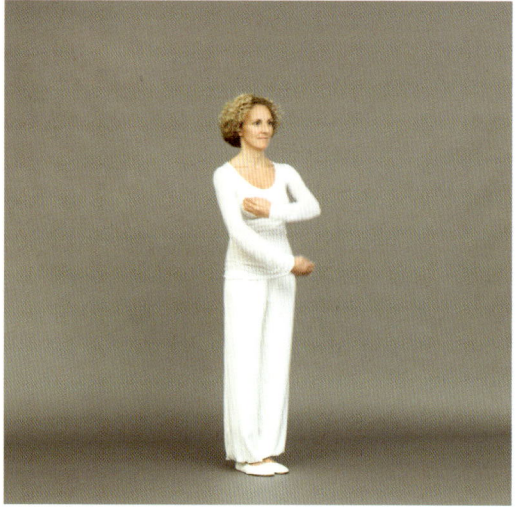

3 Gently lower your arms back to your sides.

Consonant Exercises

B

Leg movement

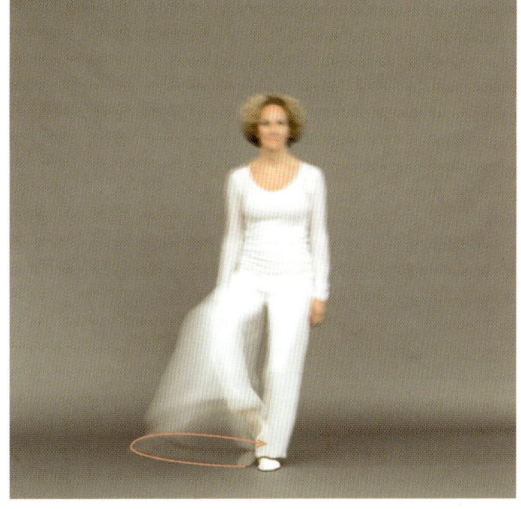

1 Stand firm with your knees relaxed. Imitate the enclosing arm movements you did, but this time with your legs: first with your right, then left leg. Take a step forwards between each movement.

Combined movements I

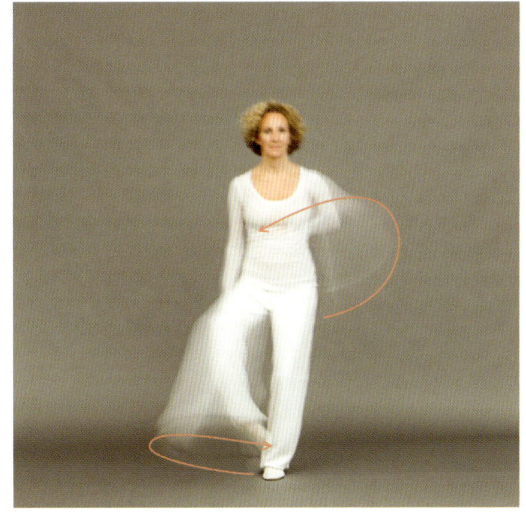

1 With your right leg and left arm, perform an enveloping B movement and step forwards. Now do the same with your left leg and right arm. Repeat this several times.

Consonant Exercises

Combined movements II

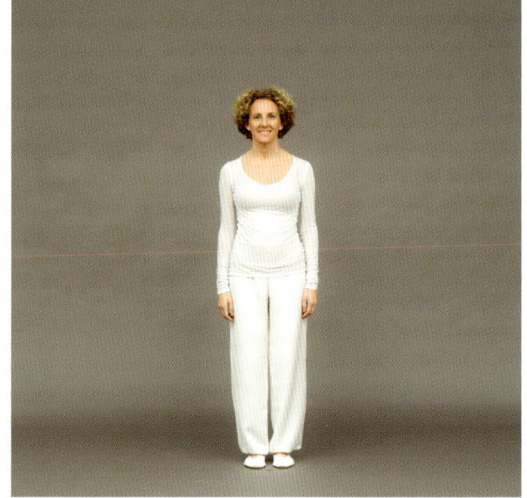

1 Stand upright. Feel a connection to the earth with your feet. Keep your knees loose and breathe calmly. Place your arms by your sides. Rest your gaze on the horizon. The movement impulse will emanate from your shoulder blades.

Consonant Exercises

B

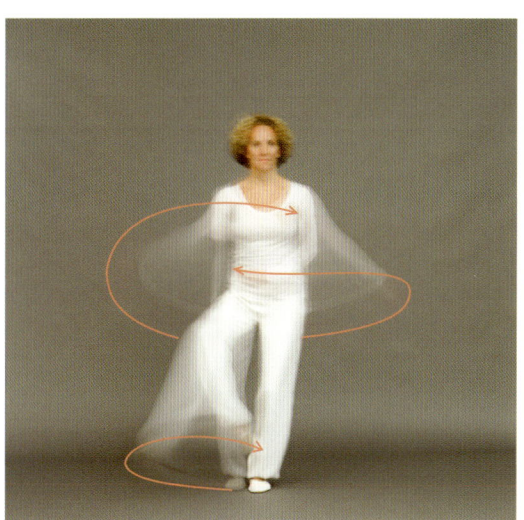

2 With your right leg and both arms simultaneously, perform an enclosing B movement. Step forward as you do so. Repeat with your left leg and both arms.

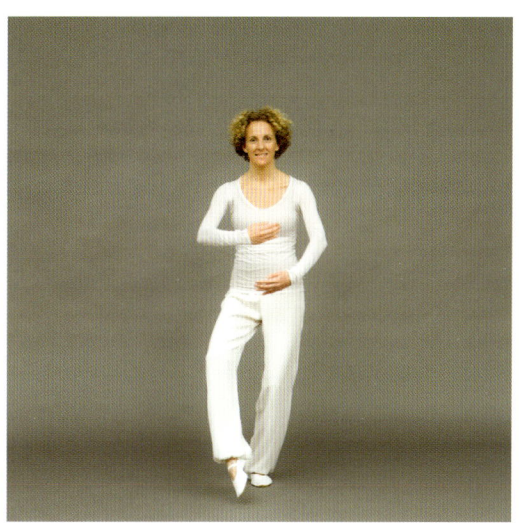

3 After your final repetition, release your arms to your sides.

Tips

✱ Repeat the sequence for a few minutes until you tire.

✱ Speed up the movement sequence as you go.

✱ Keep your inner picture in mind and move within it.

✱ Allow the consonant to work within you for a while after you finish.

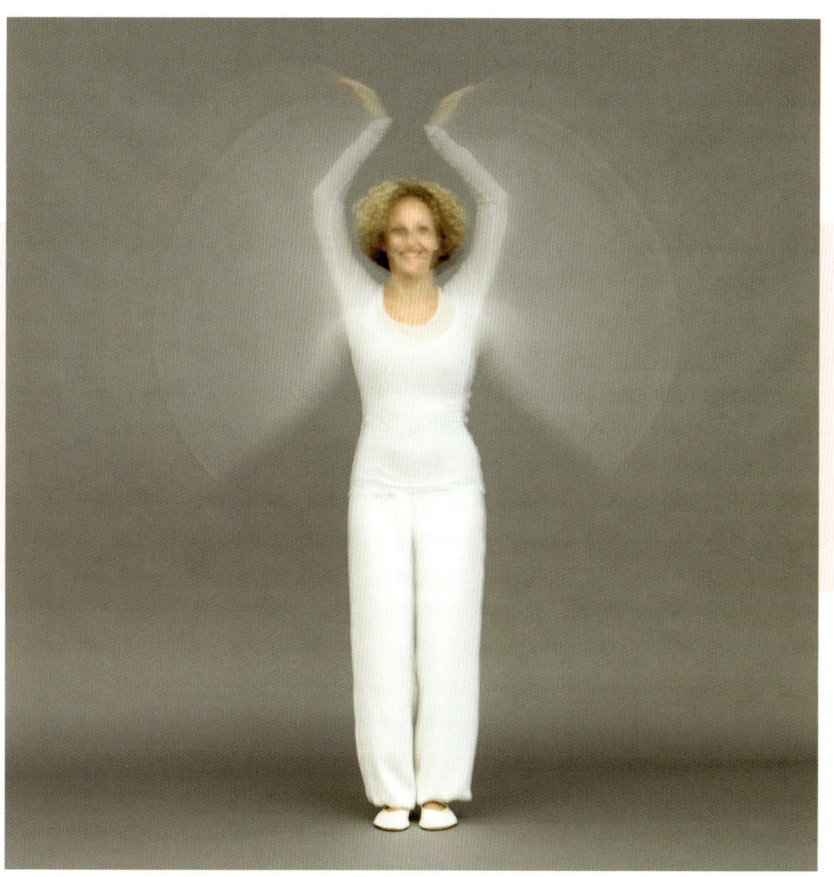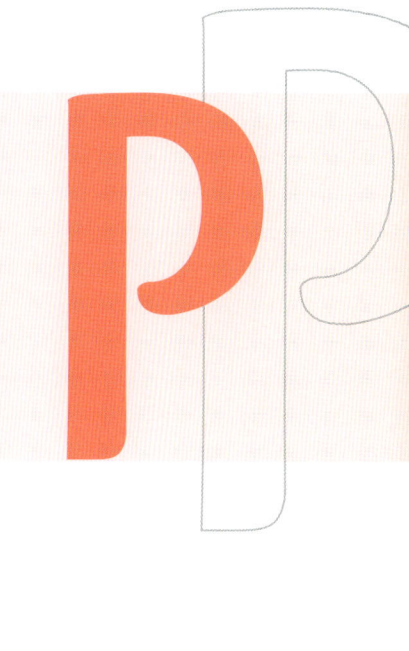

Enveloping and drawing in

- Encourages firmness, calm, consolidation
- Helps with breathing
- Supports organ growth
- Protects a sense of self
- Has a qualitative affinity with B

Inner picture Imagine drawing something protective over you, like a mantle, cloak or blanket. With each repetition of the gesture, the layer becomes denser.

Consonant Exercises

Arm movement

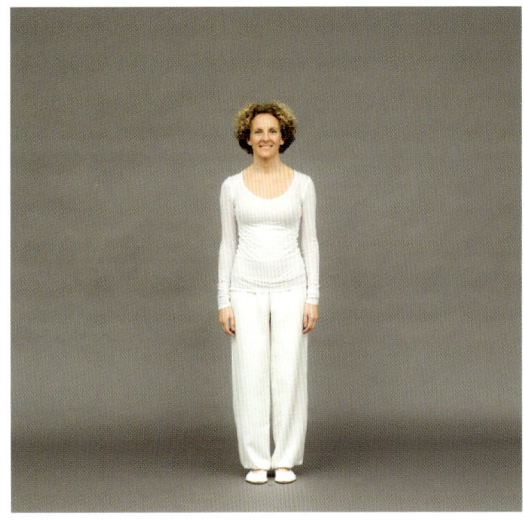

1 Stand upright. Feel a connection to the earth with your feet. Keep your knees loose and breathe calmly. Place your arms by your sides. Rest your gaze on the horizon. The movement impulse will emanate from your shoulder blades.

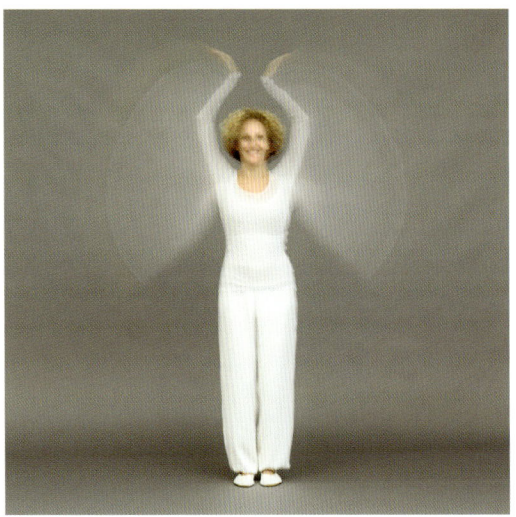

2 Raise your arms above your head, with palms facing downwards like a preying mantis.

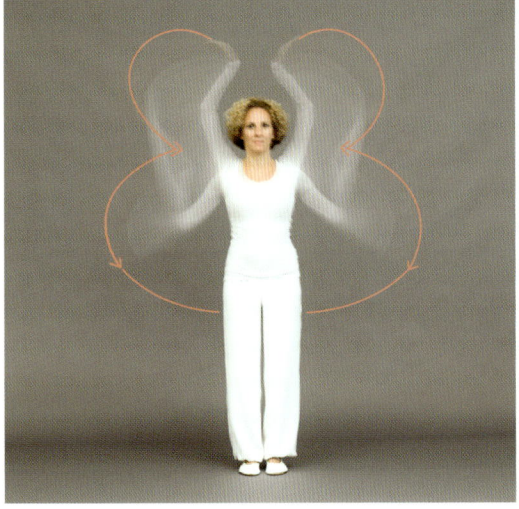

3 Let your arms curve out and around in an arc to meet at your sides.

Consonant Exercises

P

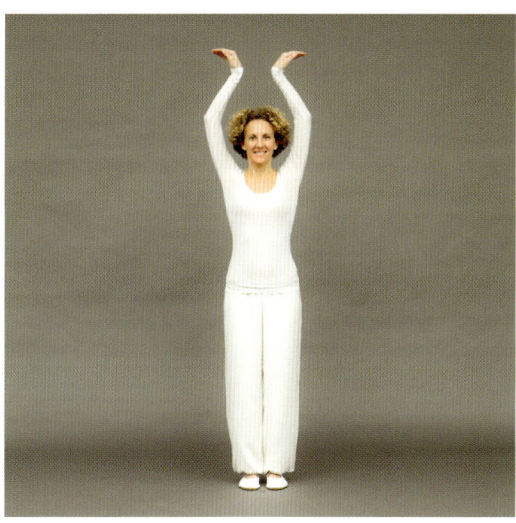

4 Repeat the movement three times at different levels: from above your head

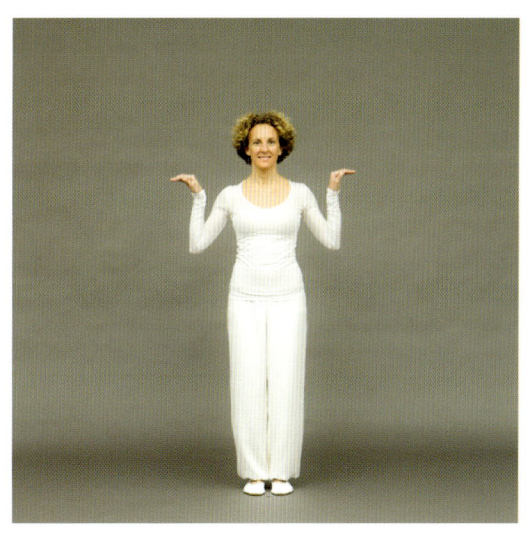

From shoulder level

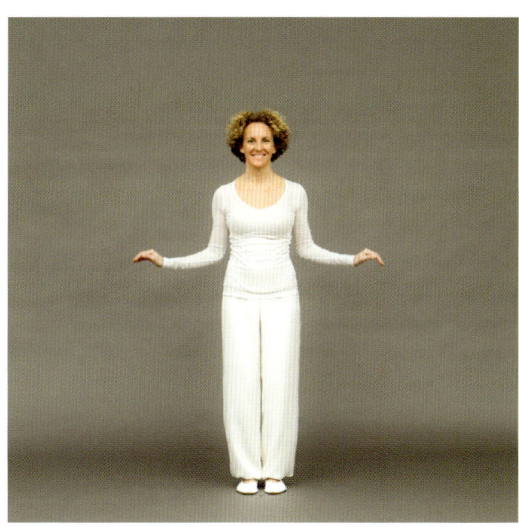

From the hips

Consonant Exercises

Leg movement

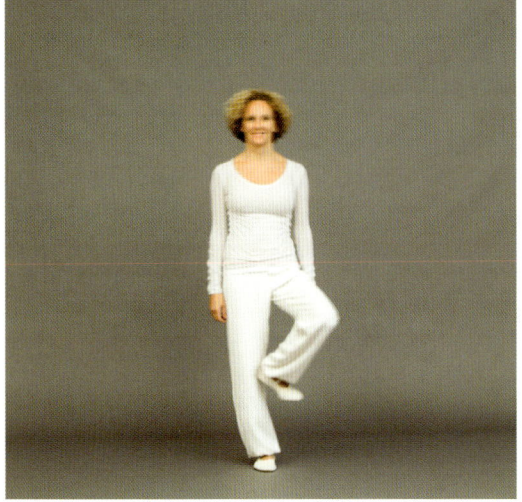

1 Bend your left leg and draw the heel in to meet your right knee. Then gently lower your foot and take a step forward as you do so. Complete the action with your right leg and walk forwards as you repeat.

Consonant Exercises

Combined movements

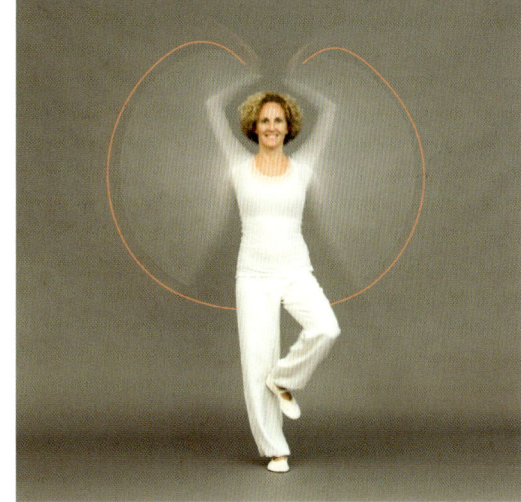

1 Make the P gesture with your arms (either at one or at three different levels) while moving your legs at the same time. Speed up the movement sequence as you go.

Tips

- Repeat the sequence for a few minutes until you tire.
- Keep your inner picture in mind and move within it
- Allow the consonant to work within you for a while after you finish.
- Variation: the P movement can also be done with both legs simultaneously, the heels touching as you do a little jump in the air.

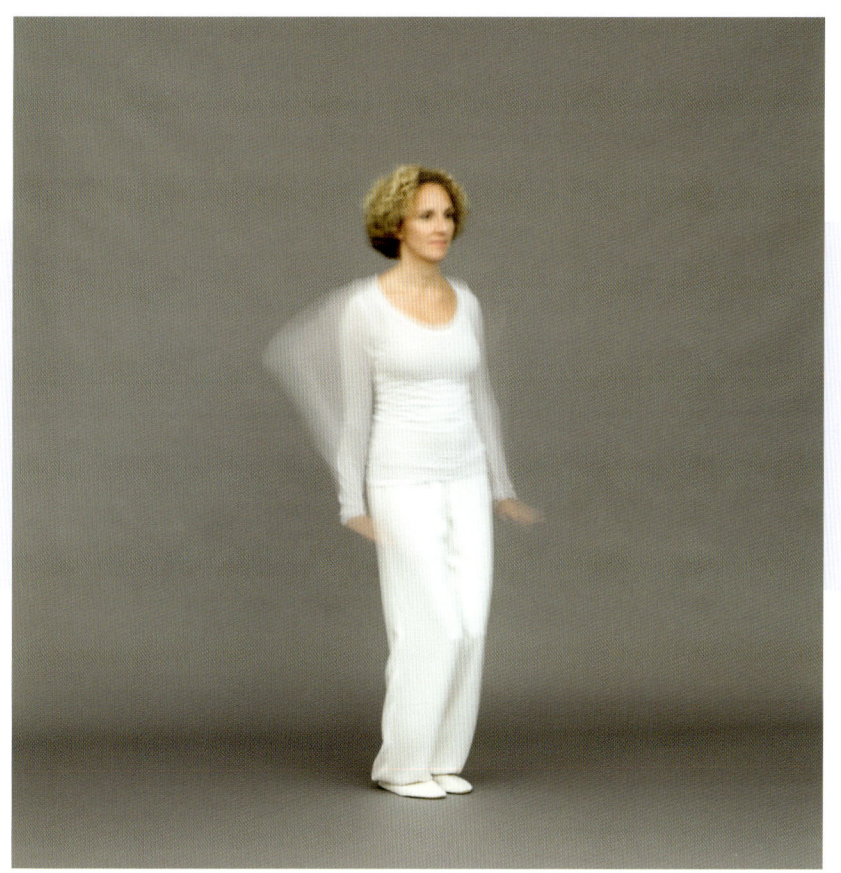
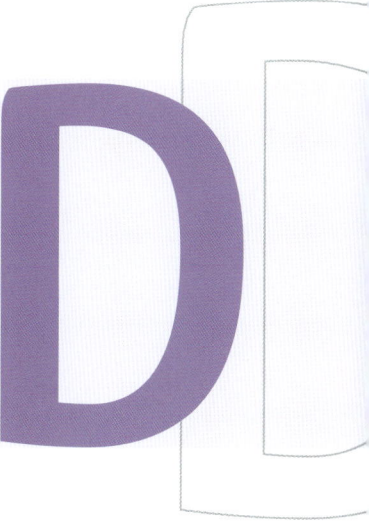

Gently descending

- Encourages a sense of grounding, strength, calm
- Soothes and consolidates the soul
- Helps to inhabit the body and stand against the earth's gravity
- Stimulates metabolic processes
- Has a qualitative affinity with T

Inner picture Imagine you are letting warm sunrays stream from your hands to permeate your whole body from above downwards.

Consonant Exercises

Arm movement

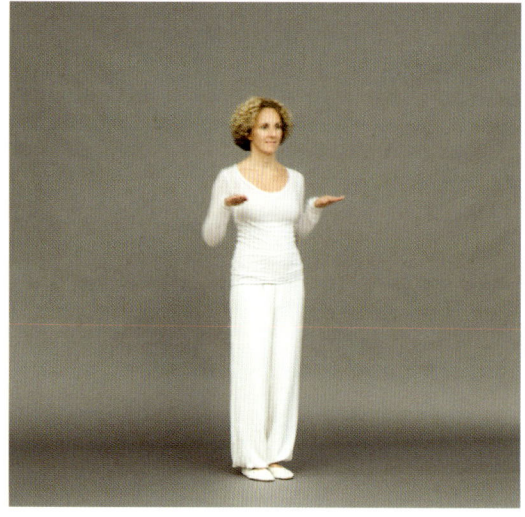

1 Stand upright. Feel a connection to the earth with your feet. Keep your knees loose and breathe calmly. Place your hands at chest height, pointing forwards with the palms facing down. Rest your gaze on the horizon. The movement impulse will emanate from your shoulder blades.

Consonant Exercises

D

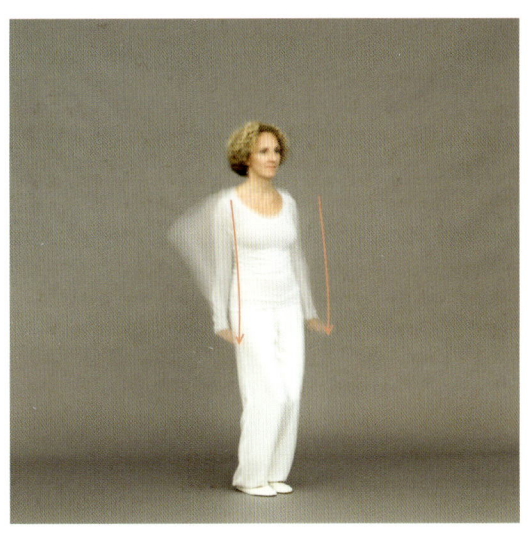 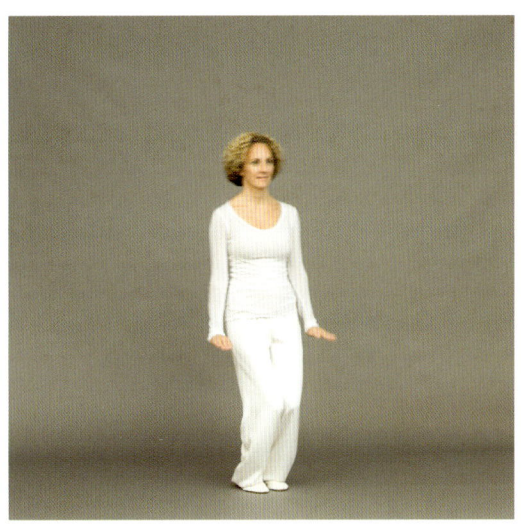

2 Gently lower your hands down either side of your body, keeping the palms level, bending your knees as you go.

3 Release back to a neutral standing position.

Tip

☼ Feel the resistance of air as you push through it with the palms of your hands.

Consonant Exercises

Combined movements I

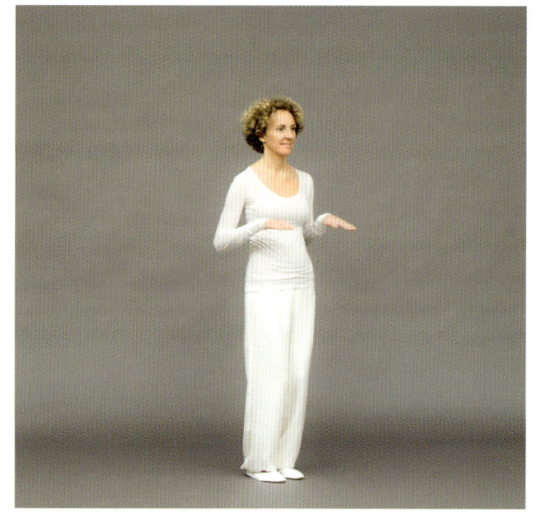

1 Begin with your hands at chest height, as you did in the arm movement. Lower your hands gently to diaphragm level. Lightly bend your knees and hop.

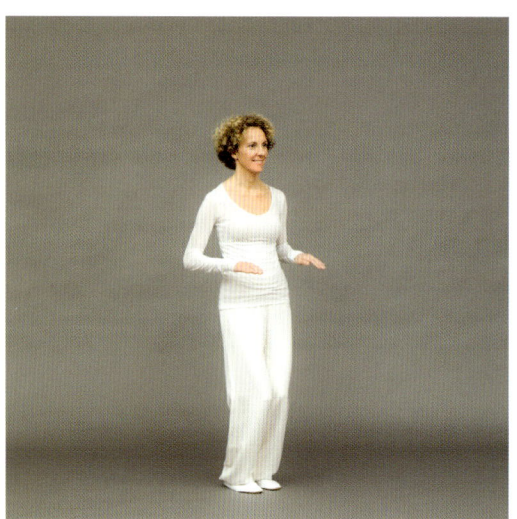

2 Bring the hands upwards again then lower them gently to hip level. Hop again, bending your knees slightly more this time.

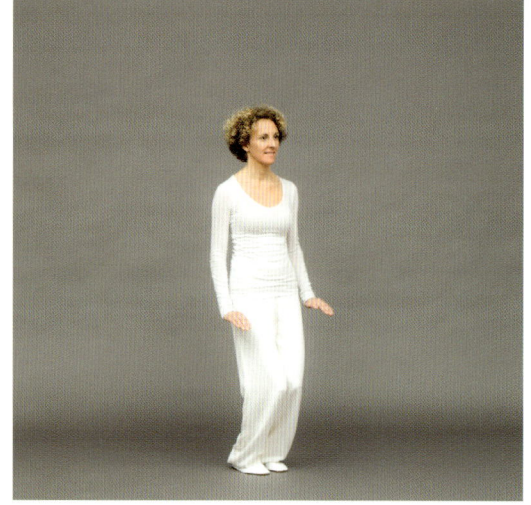

3 Bring the hands upwards again then lower them until they are level with your upper thigh. Bend the knees deeper and hop again. Repeat the sequence as many times as you like.

Consonant Exercises

Combined movements II

Tips

☼ Repeat the sequence – either hopping or stepping – for a few minutes until you tire.

☼ Keep your inner picture in mind and move within it.

☼ Allow the consonant to work within you for a while after you finish.

D

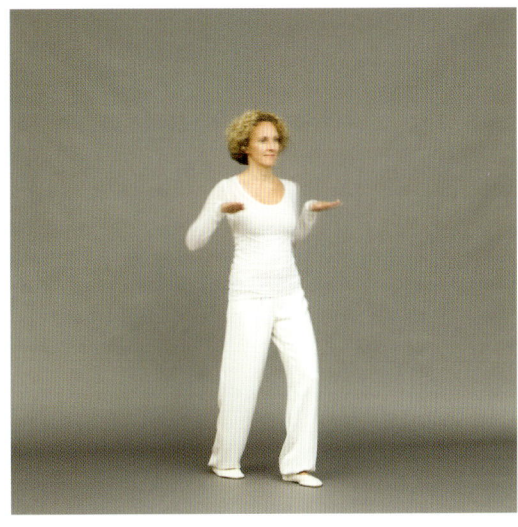

1 Begin with your hands at chest height, as you did in the arm movement. Lower your hands gently to diaphragm level. Bending your knees, take one step forward with your left leg.

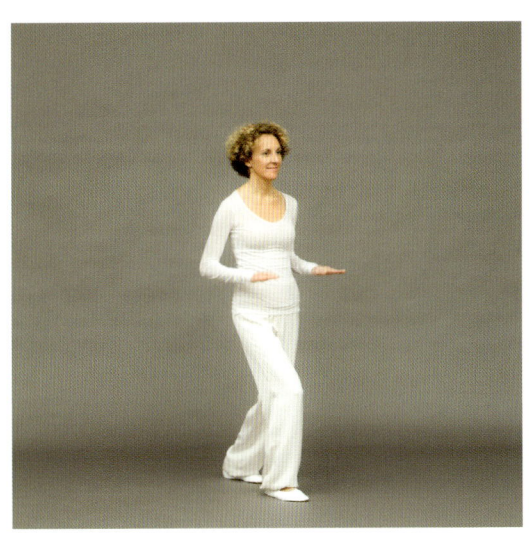

2 Swing the hands upwards again then lower them gently to hip level. As you do so, bend the knees slightly take one more step forwards with your right leg this time.

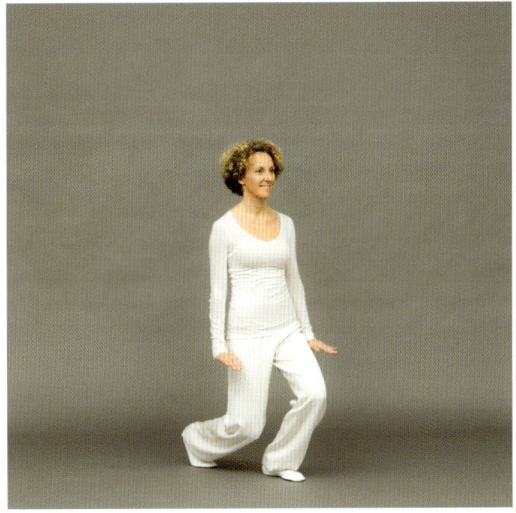

3 Swing the hands upwards again then lower them to upper thigh level. Take another step and bend the knees as low as you can.

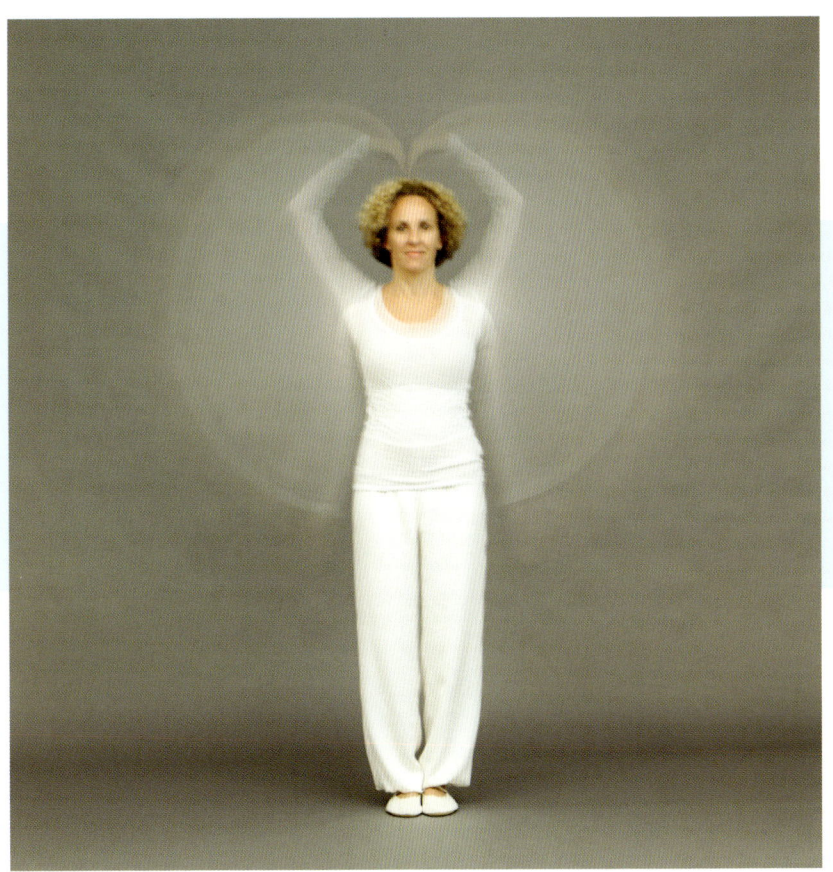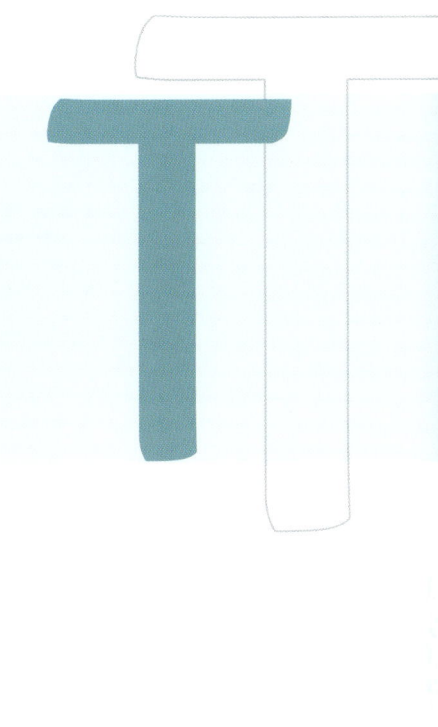

Inwardly radiating

- Encourages centeredness, strength, stimulation, order
- Heartens and warms the body
- Draws us up to our full height
- Nurtures a stronger self-awareness
- Has a qualitative affinity with D

Inner picture Imagine you are receiving the broad expanse of the heavens into your arms. Feel the strengthening powers of nature streaming down through you from your head to your toes.

Consonant Exercises

Arm movement

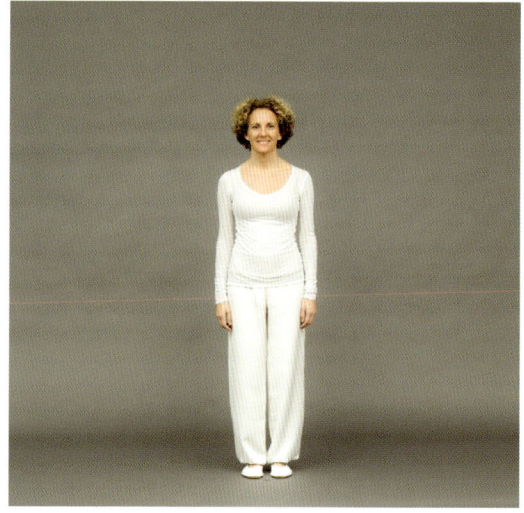

1 Stand upright. Feel a connection to the earth with your feet. Keep your knees loose and breathe calmly. Place your hands at chest height, pointing forwards with the palms facing down. Rest your gaze on the horizon. The movement impulse will emanate from your shoulder blades.

Consonant Exercises

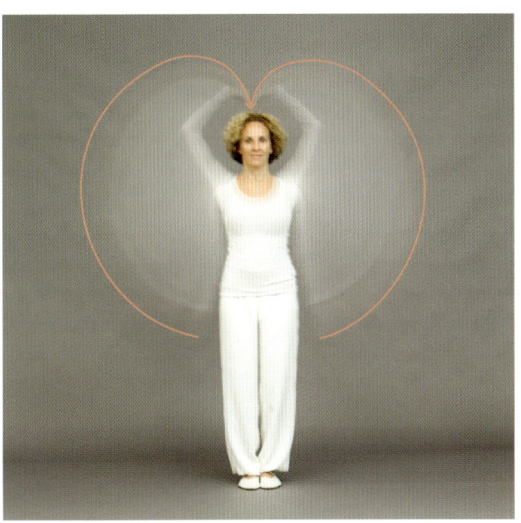

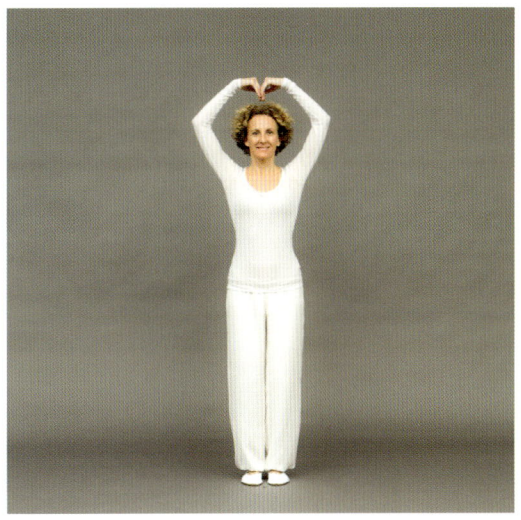

2 Sweep your arms up in a wide arc and bring your hands together above the head. Your fingers should meet inwards like the top of a heart.

3 Release back to your neutral standing position.

Tip

☼ Cup your palms upwards as you raise them, as if you are collecting light to pour back down onto your head.

Consonant Exercises

Leg movement

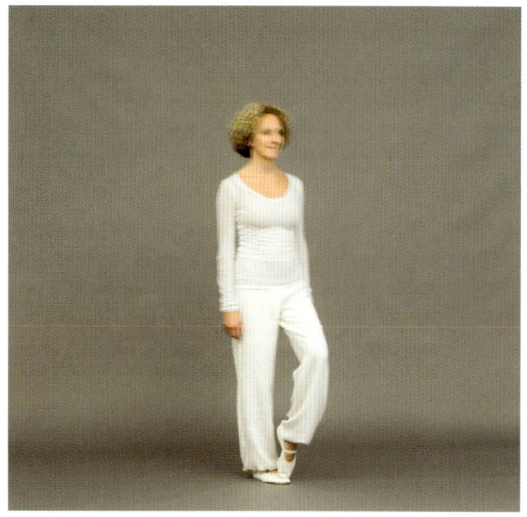

1 Point your left toes on top of your right toes, and sense them connecting. Then take a step forwards with your left leg. Repeat with your right leg.

Consonant Exercises

Combined movement

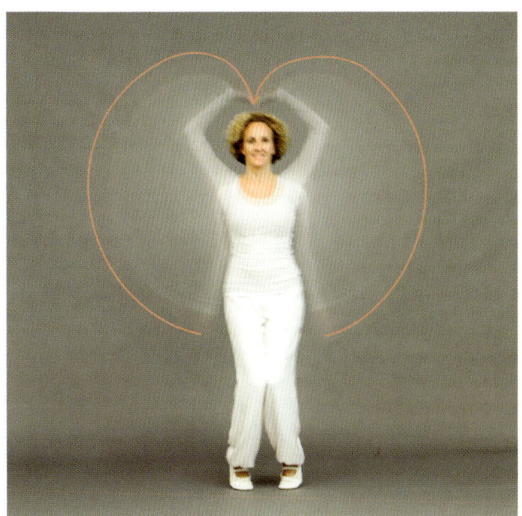
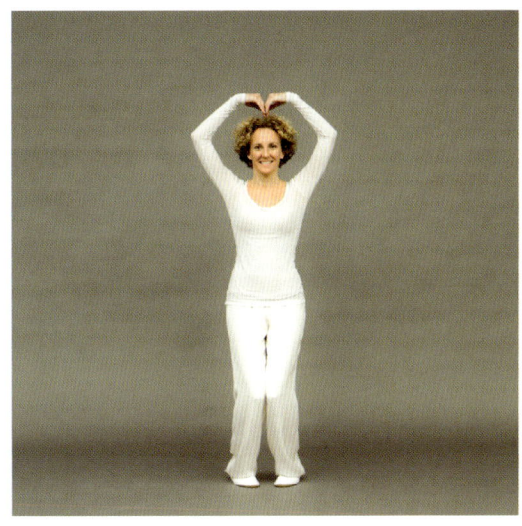

1 Begin the arm movement as instructed on page 78. When your hands meet over your head, bring your knees inwards (as if to form an X with your legs) and rise onto your toes. You can also add a little forward jump to advance the movement.

2 Place your heels back on the ground and release.

Tips

- ✧ Repeat each sequence – either standing or jumping – for a few minutes until you tire.
- ✧ Keep your inner picture in mind and feel the rays shining into your head from your hands all the way down to your feet.
- ✧ Allow the consonant to work within you for a while after you finish.

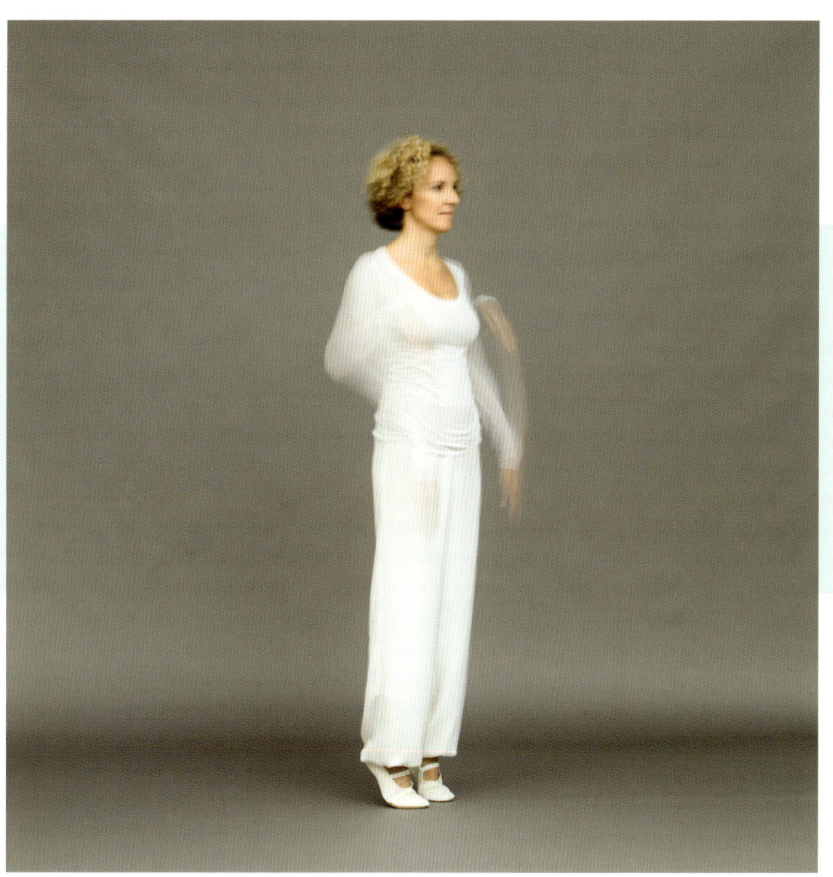
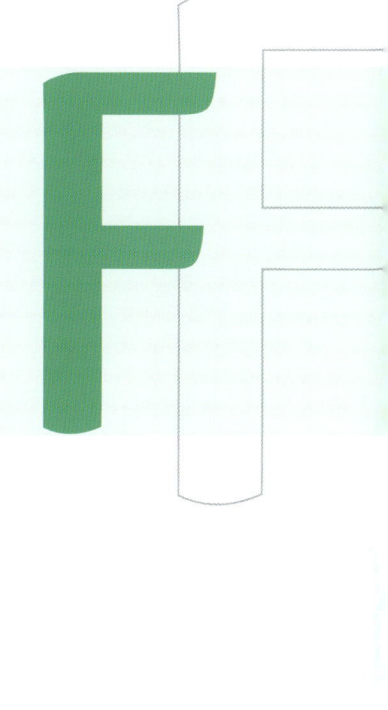

Airborne intention

- Encourages warmth, resolve, receptiveness
- An outwardly directed impulse

Inner picture Imagine you are energetically fanning a fire. Then stand back and leave it to glow.

Consonant Exercises

Arm movement

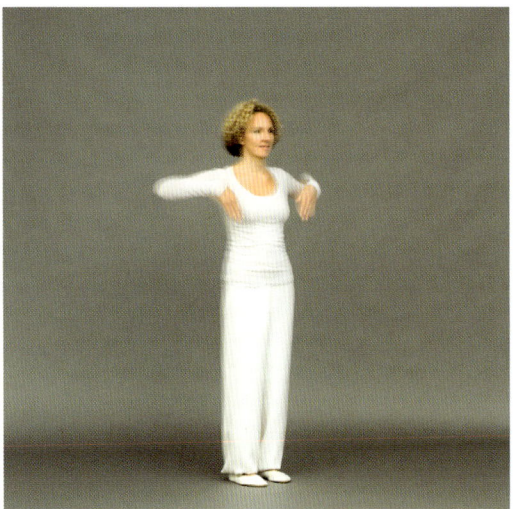 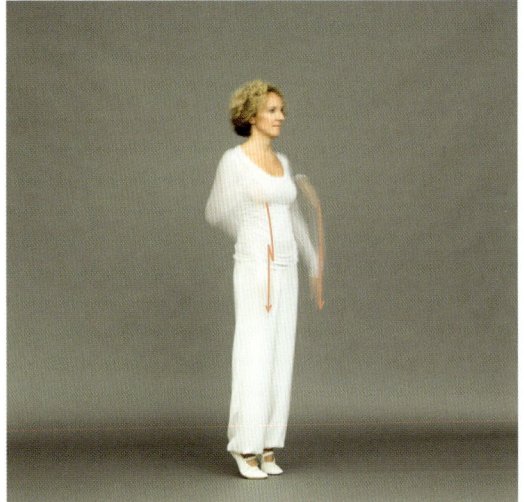

1 Stand upright. Feel a connection to the earth with your feet. Keep your knees loose and breathe calmly. Place your arms at chest height, elbows out, hands pointing downwards. Rest your gaze on the horizon. The movement impulse will emanate from your shoulder blades.

2 First make a slight downward movement with your arms, pull back slightly and then push further downwards again. Leap onto your toes as you do so.

Tips

- ✧ Repeat the sequence for a few minutes until you tire.
- ✧ Keep your inner picture in mind and move within it, streaming air out in front of you.
- ✧ Allow the consonant to work within you for a while after you finish.

Consonant Exercises

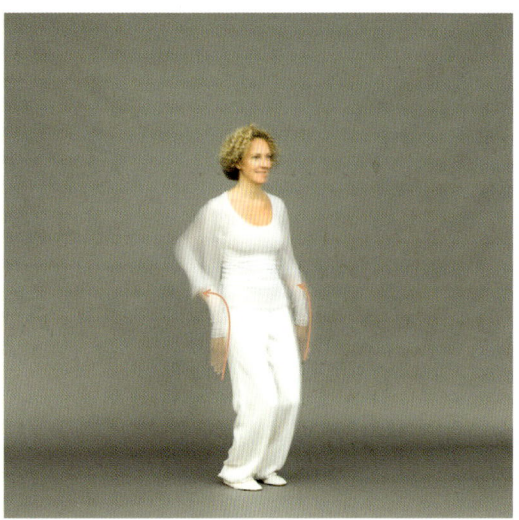 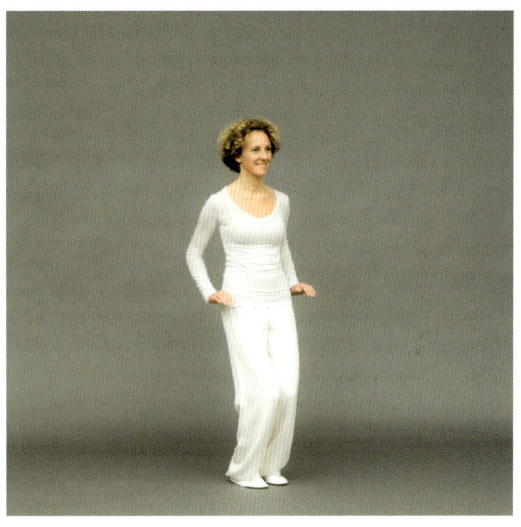

3 Let your arms drop by your sides and lead them back with bent elbows to rest at hip level. Sink back onto your heels and bend your knees slightly.

4 Rest here, then release.

Leg movement

Tip

☼ Perform your arm and leg movements together simultaneously to walk forwards with these powerful gestures.

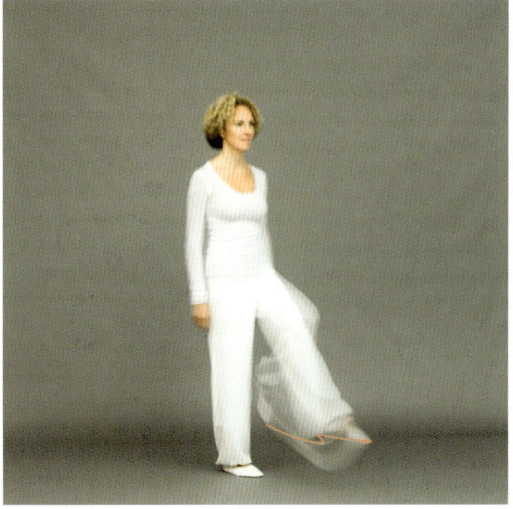

1 Imitate the arm movement by moving your left leg forwards in a two-part, lightly pushing motion. Then lower your foot and take a step. Do the same with the other leg, and repeat.

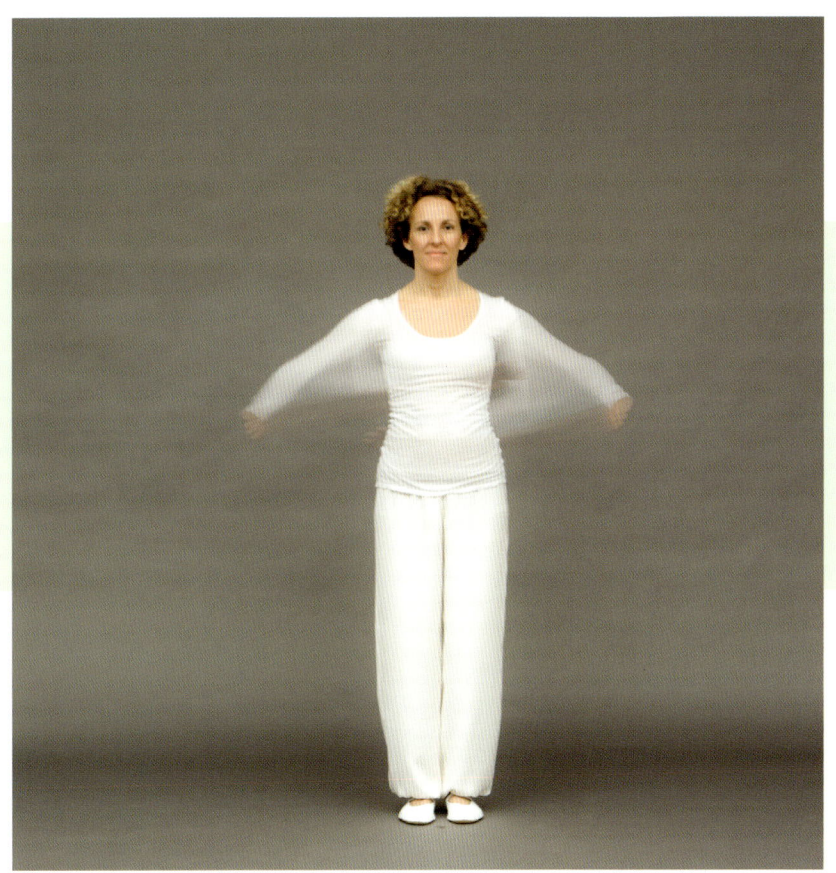
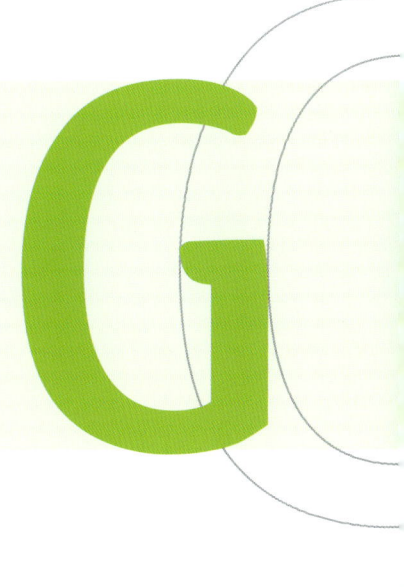

Calmly repelling

- ☼ Encourages expansion from within
- ☼ Creates space
- ☼ Stimulates the digestive system
- ☼ Helps define the self in relation to our surroundings
- ☼ Has a qualitative affinity with K

Inner picture   Imagine the light in your own life as a candle that needs more air to burn. Expand the space inside you and fill it with brightness.

Consonant Exercises

Arm movement I

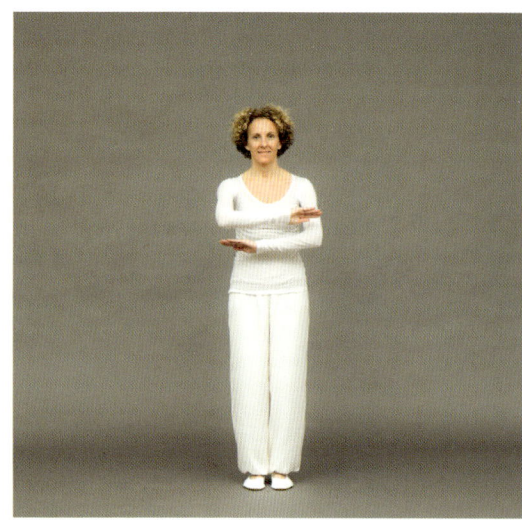

1 Stand upright. Feel a connection to the earth with your feet. Keep your knees loose and breathe calmly. Place your arms at chest height, crossing over each other but not touching. Rest your gaze on the horizon. The movement impulse will emanate from your shoulder blades.

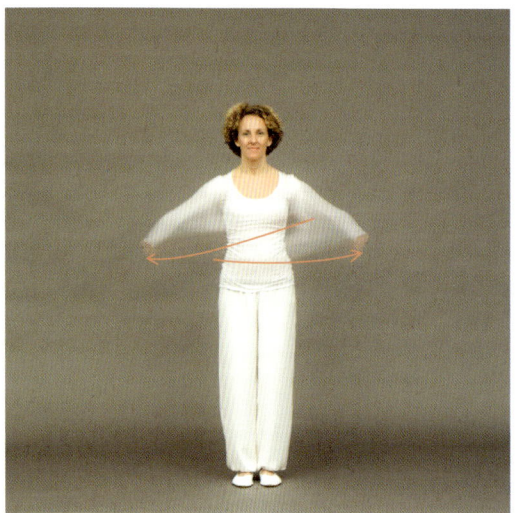

2 Make a calm movement outwards with both arms, creating space from within.

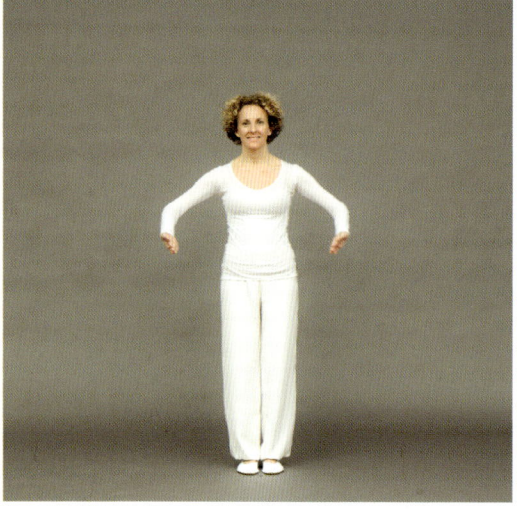

3 Release your arms down to your sides.

Consonant Exercises

Arm movement II

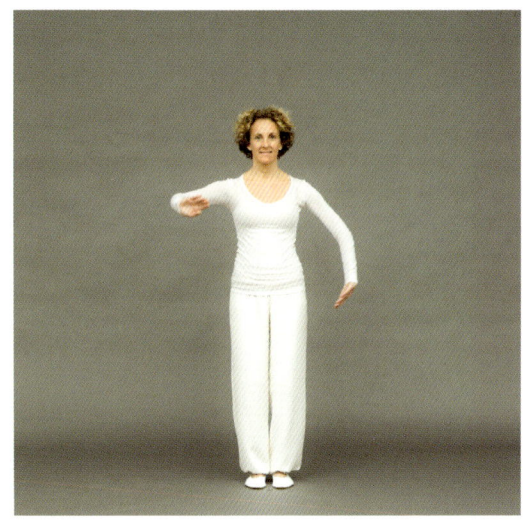

1 The G arm gesture can also be done with asymmetrical arm movements, moving outwards to fill the whole space as you repeat.

Consonant Exercises

Combined movements

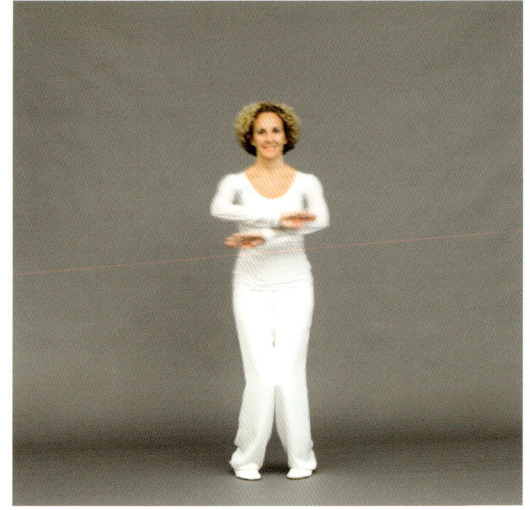

1 Stand upright. Feel a connection to the earth with your feet. Keep your knees loose and breathe calmly. Place your arms at chest height, crossing over each other but not touching. Bring your knees in to meet, heels pointing outwards. Rest your gaze on the horizon. The movement impulse will emanate from your shoulder blades.

Consonant Exercises

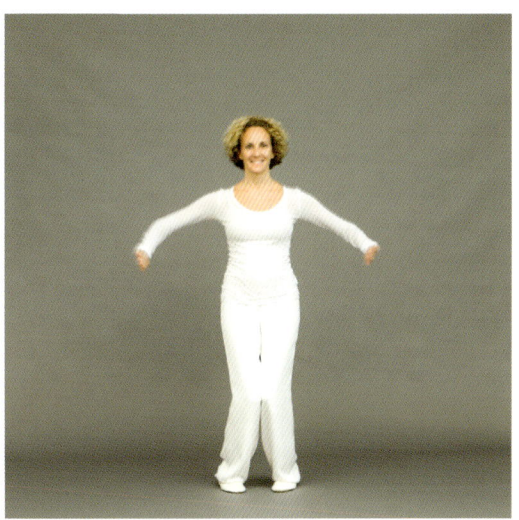

2 Move your arms as you did in either variation on pages 88-89. As you do so, jump forward, keeping your legs in an X shape.

3 Release back to a neutral standing pose.

G

Tips

✧ Repeat the sequence – either symmetrically or asymmetrically – for a few minutes until you tire.

✧ Keep your inner picture in mind and move within the space you have created, protected from the outer world.

✧ Allow the consonant to work within you for a while after you finish.

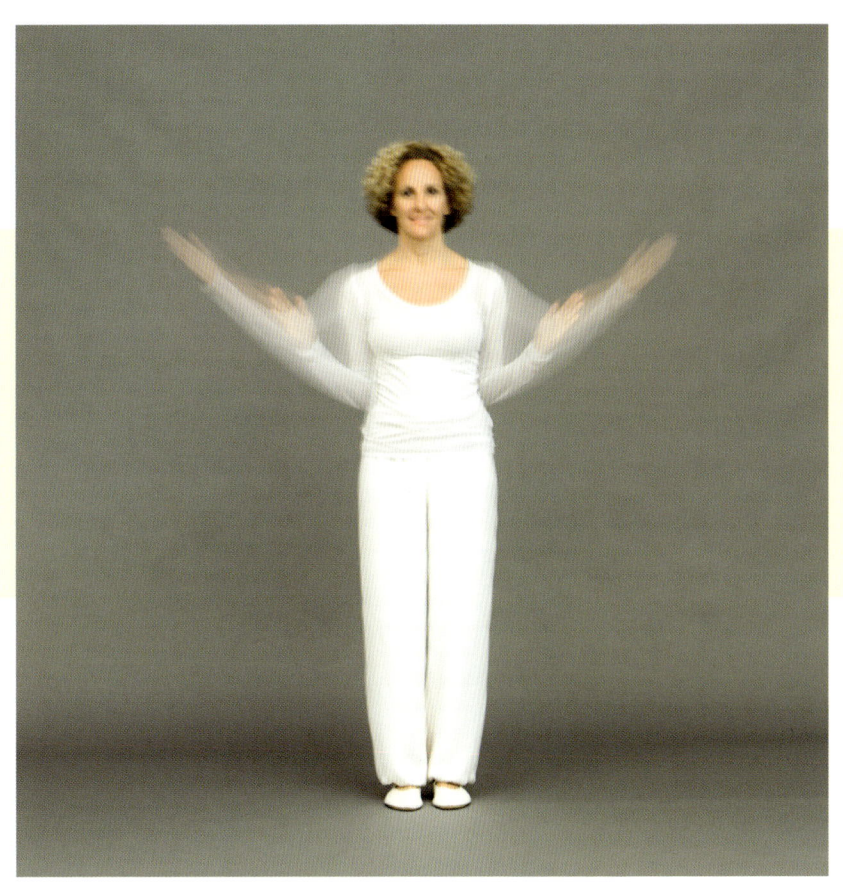
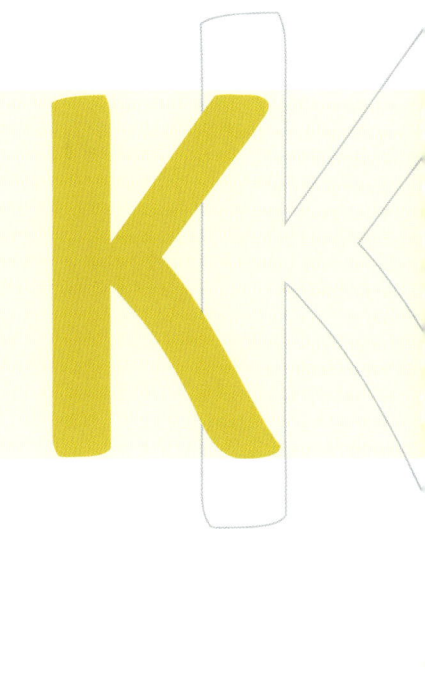

Energetically repelling

- Encourages strength, outward impulses
- Pushes away negative influences
- Stimulates digestion
- Has a qualitative affinity with G

Inner picture Imagine chopping wood with an axe, but rather than coming to a standstill after this strong impact, everything goes on lightly reverberating.

Consonant Exercises

Arm movement

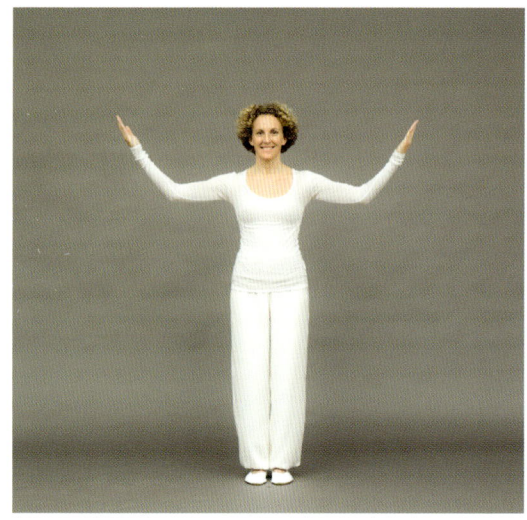

1 Stand upright. Feel a connection to the earth with your feet. Keep your knees loose and breathe calmly. Raise your arms in a wide-open gesture. Rest your gaze on the horizon. The movement impulse will emanate from your shoulder blades.

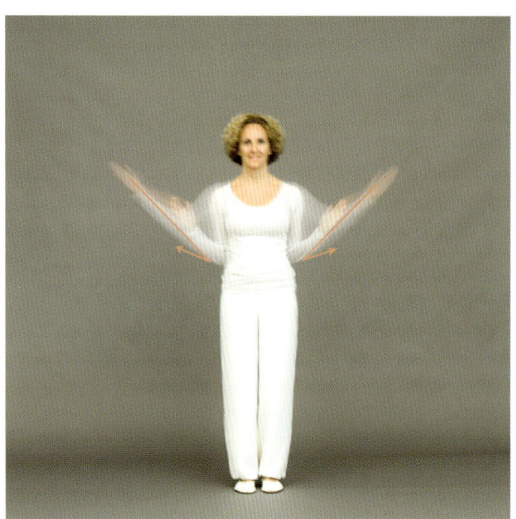

2 Make an repelling movement in front of you, palms facing upwards. Let the arms spring back a little after this.

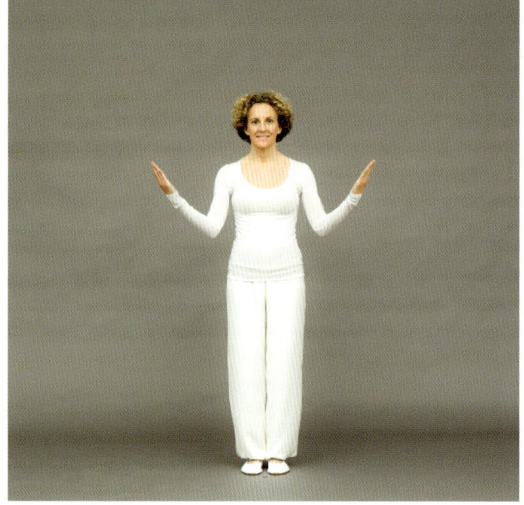

3 And release back to a neutral pose.

Consonant Exercises

Combined movement

Tips

☼ Keep your energetic inner picture in mind and move within it.

☼ Allow the consonant to work within you for a while after you finish.

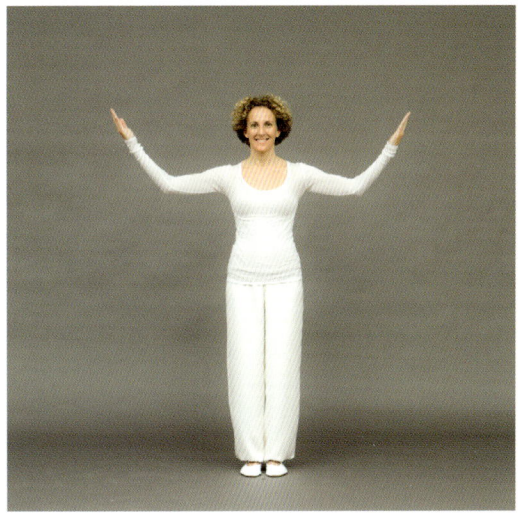

1 Stand upright. Feel a connection to the earth with your feet. Keep your knees loose and breathe calmly. Raise your arms in a wide-open gesture. Rest your gaze on the horizon. The movement impulse will emanate from your shoulder blades.

K

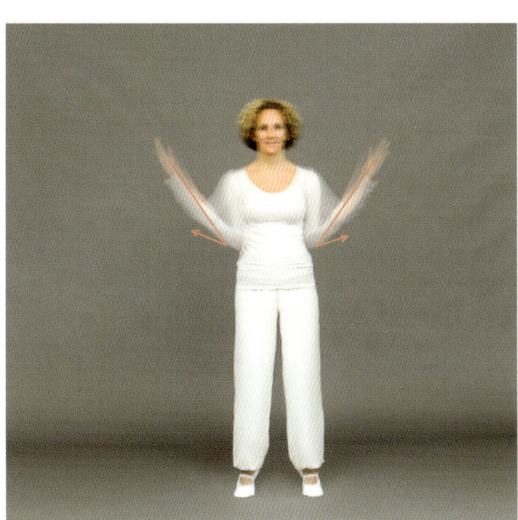

2 Make the arm movement from page 94 while bouncing lightly onto your toes, legs slightly apart. Then lower your heels.

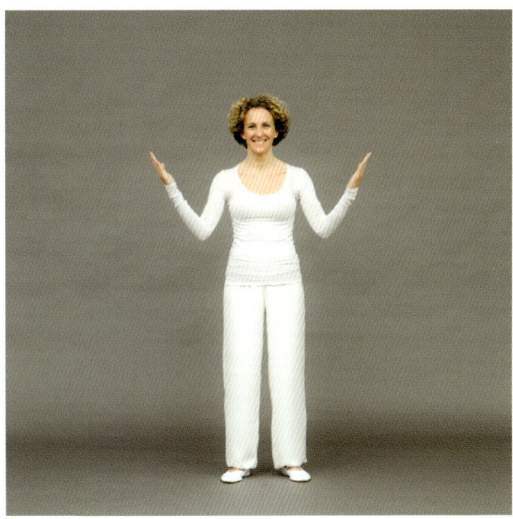

3 And release back to a neutral pose. Repeat as you wish.

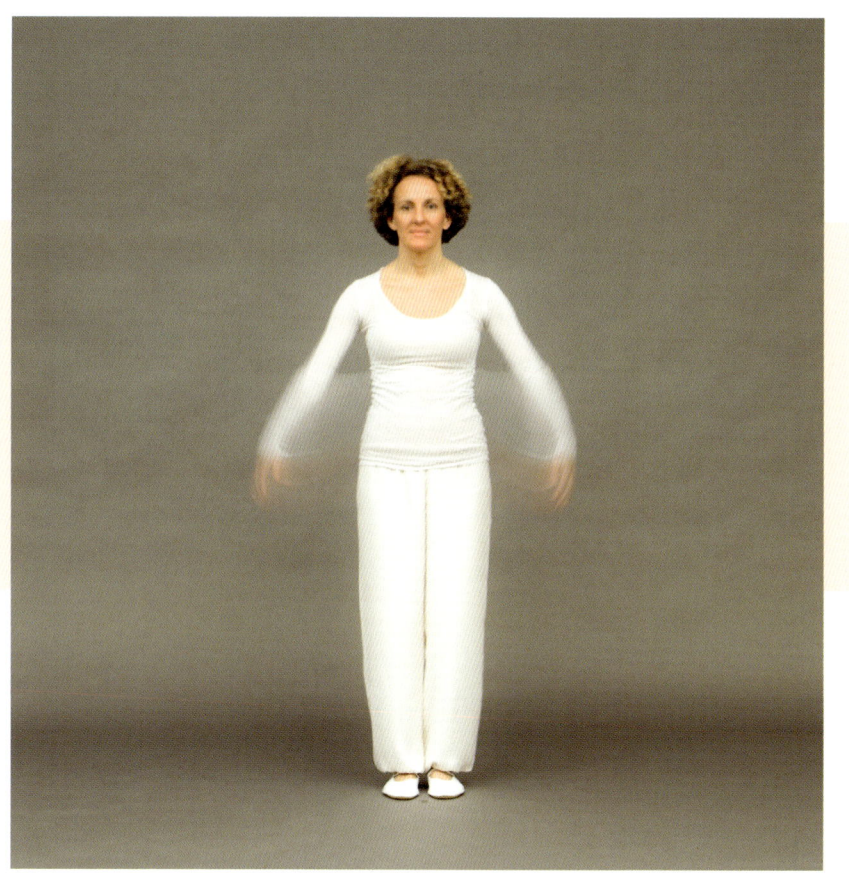
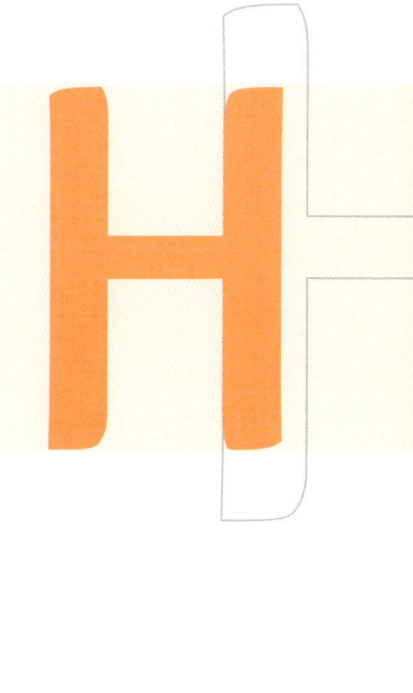

Broadening and freeing

- ☼ Encourages release, lightness, expansion
- ☼ Helps to stop us from hardening
- ☼ Frees us from burden

Inner picture Imagine your inner space widening from the centre outwards, beyond the limits of your body, but without vanishing into the periphery.

Consonant Exercises

Arm movement

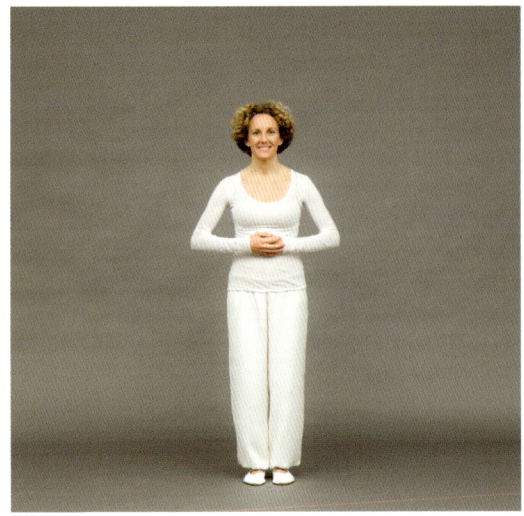

1 Stand upright. Feel a connection to the earth with your feet. Keep your knees loose and breathe calmly. Lay your hands over your diaphragm. Rest your gaze on the horizon. The movement impulse will emanate from your shoulder blades.

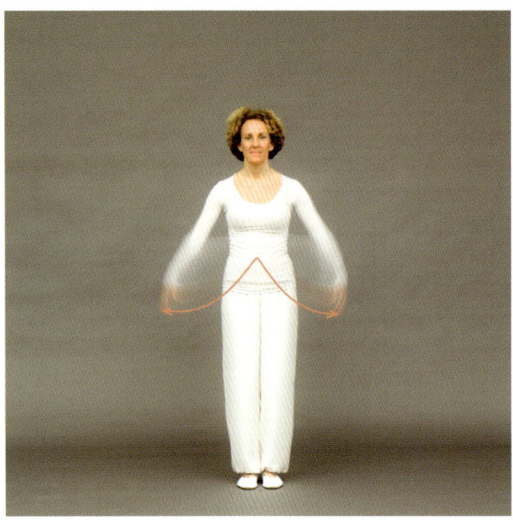

2 Make a slow, freeing sweep outwards and downwards.

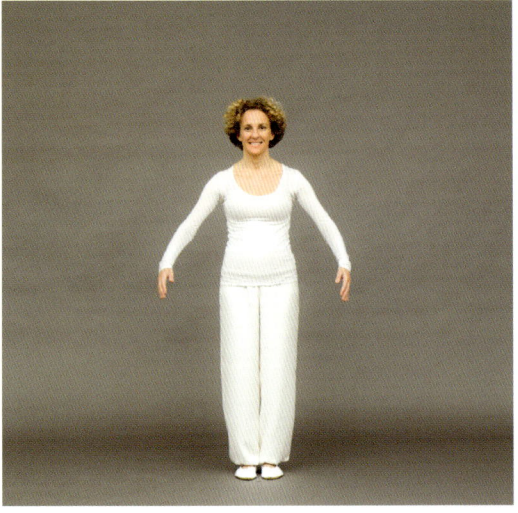

3 Come to a stop when your arms find resistance, and rest.

Consonant Exercises

Combined movement

Tips

- ☼ Keep your inner picture in mind and move within the expanding space.
- ☼ Allow the consonant to work within you for a while after you finish.

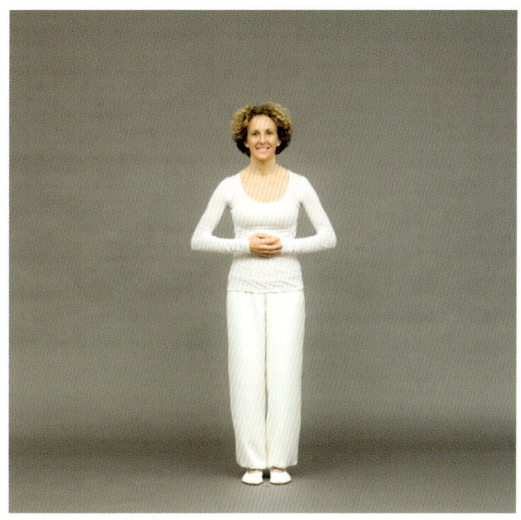

1 Stand upright. Feel a connection to the earth with your feet. Keep your knees loose and breathe calmly. Lay your hands over your diaphragm. Rest your gaze on the horizon. The movement impulse will emanate from your shoulder blades.

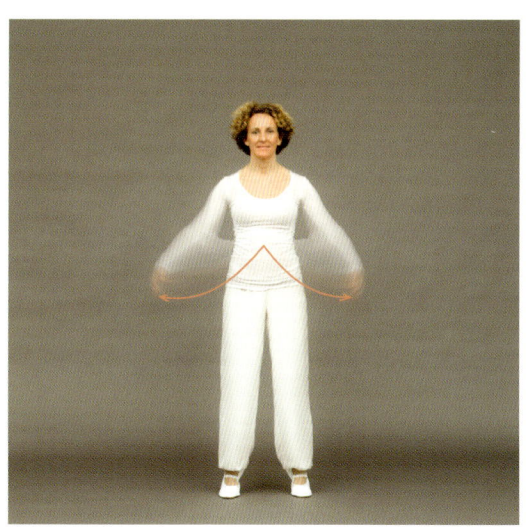

2 With your arms, make a slow, freeing movement outwards and (depending on medical indication) downwards. At the same time, leap onto your toes with slightly spread legs.

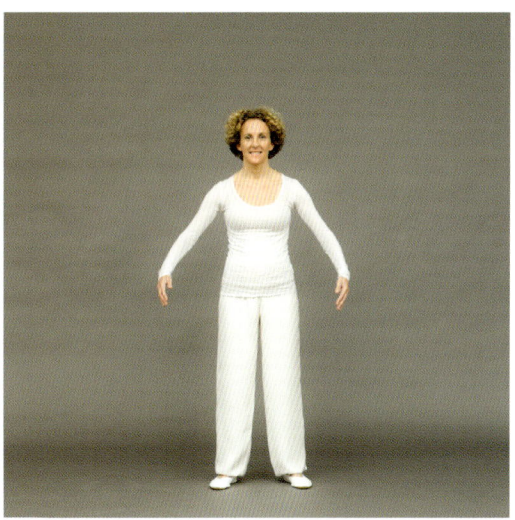

3 Slowly sink back onto your heels and release your arms to your sides. Repeat as many times as you like, resting between each jump.

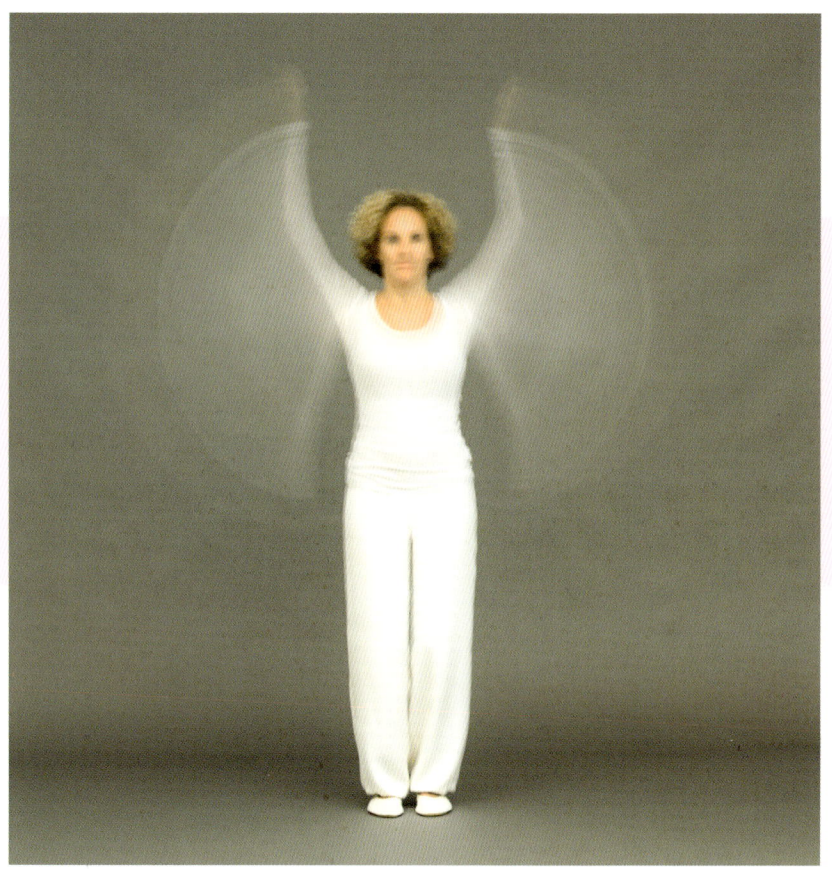

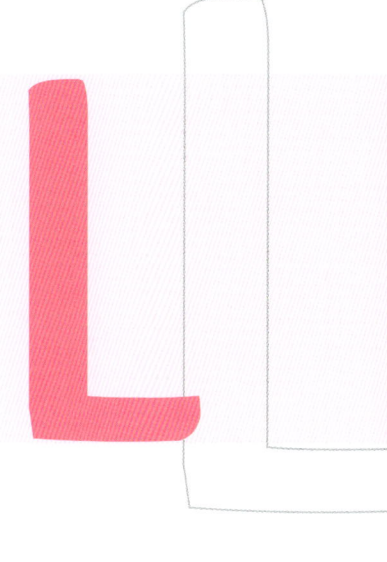

Wavelike transformation

- ☼ Encourages regulation, vitality and release
- ☼ Helps to dissolve blockages and bring flow again
- ☼ Corresponds to the lifecycle of growth and decay

Inner picture   Imagine a plant that germinates in the earth, grows towards the light of the sun, forms a flower and then lets its seed fall back to earth. Or imagine the water cycle: a spring bubbling up from the earth, evaporating into air, collecting in a cloud and returning to the earth as rain.

Consonant Exercises

Arm movement I

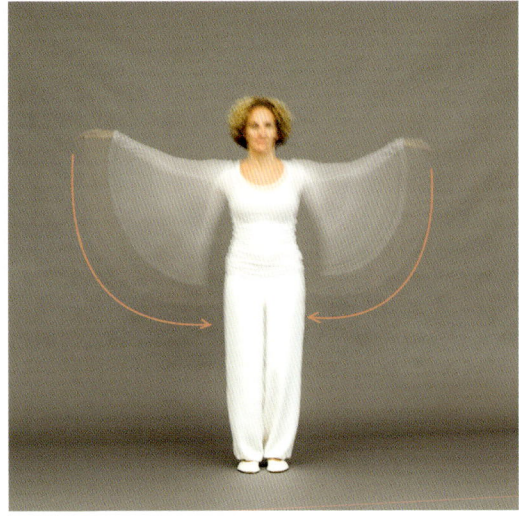

1 Stand upright. Feel a connection to the earth with your feet. Keep your knees loose and breathe calmly. Reach your arms wide on either side, level with your shoulders, palms facing downwards.

Rest your gaze on the horizon. When you feel the movement impulse, sweep your hands downwards to your sides.

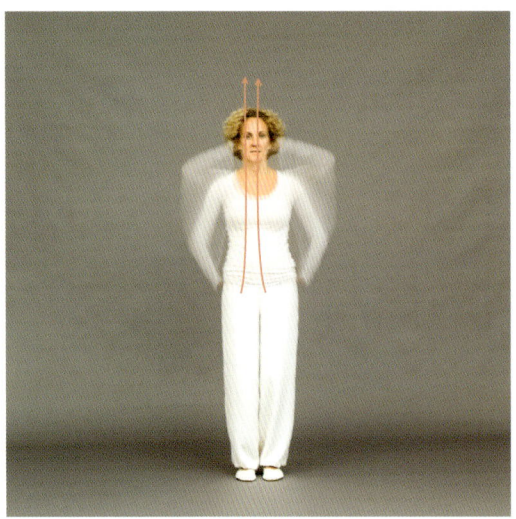

2 Cup both hands together and lift them up to head-height.

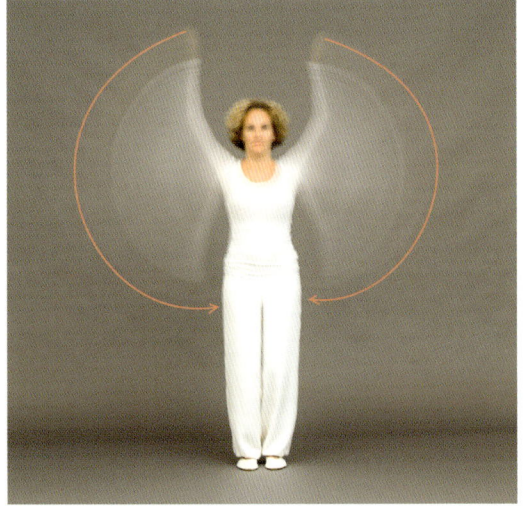

3 Continue lifting your arms over your head, separate your hands and bring your arms down to your sides in a wide circle. Keep your palms facing outwards as you do so.

Consonant Exercises

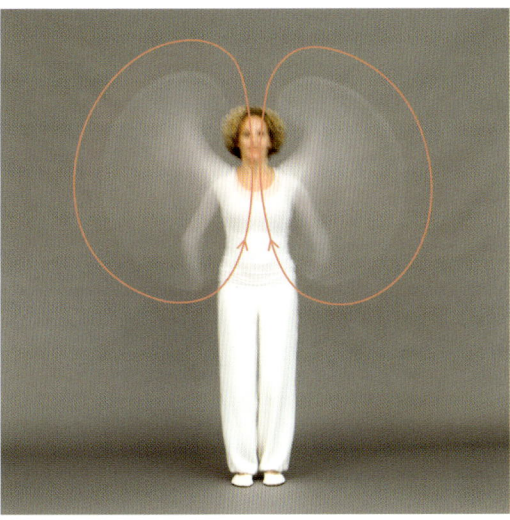

4 Repeat this circular motion by sweeping your arms up to their starting point and beginning again.

Leg movement

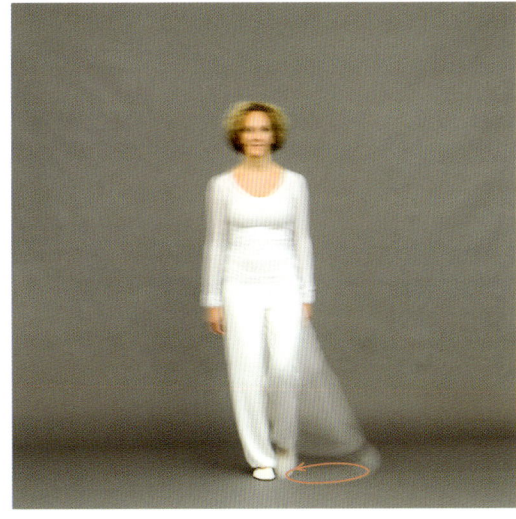

1 Make a circular movement with one leg, either clockwise or counterclockwise, then take a step forwards. Repeat the same with the other leg. This can be done backwards as well as forwards.

Consonant Exercises

Combined movement I

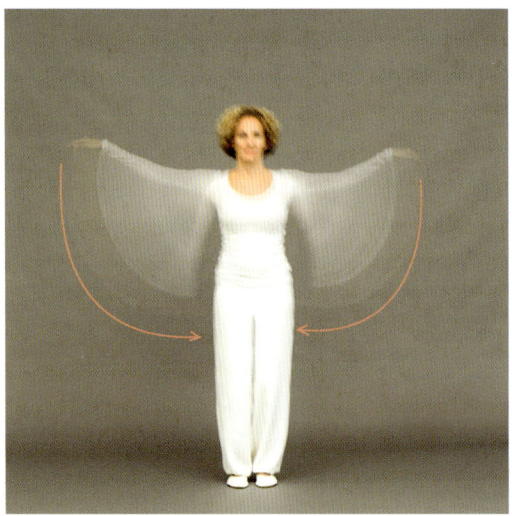

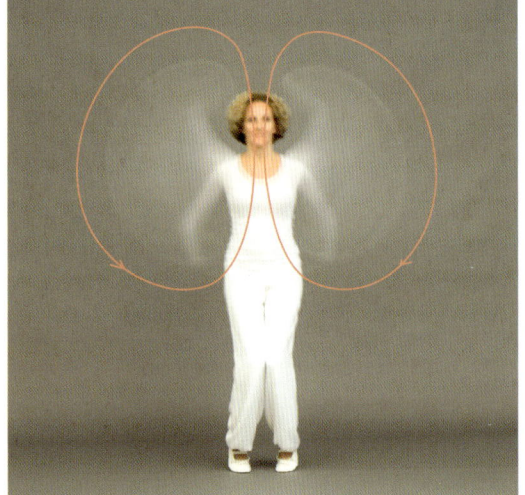

1 Perform the arm movement on page 102.

2 As the hands are moving upwards, spring onto your toes with legs in an X shape, meeting at the knees. When you release your arms, release your legs too.

Consonant Exercises

Combined movement II

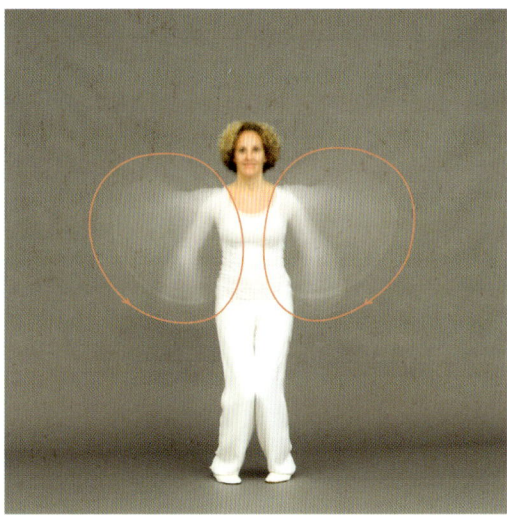

1 Perform the combined movement on page 104, but with your arms rising only to shoulder level.

Tips

- ✺ Repeat the sequence as many times as you like.
- ✺ Keep your inner picture in mind and move within its wavelike unfolding, transforming from below upwards.
- ✺ Allow the consonant to work within you for a while after you finish.

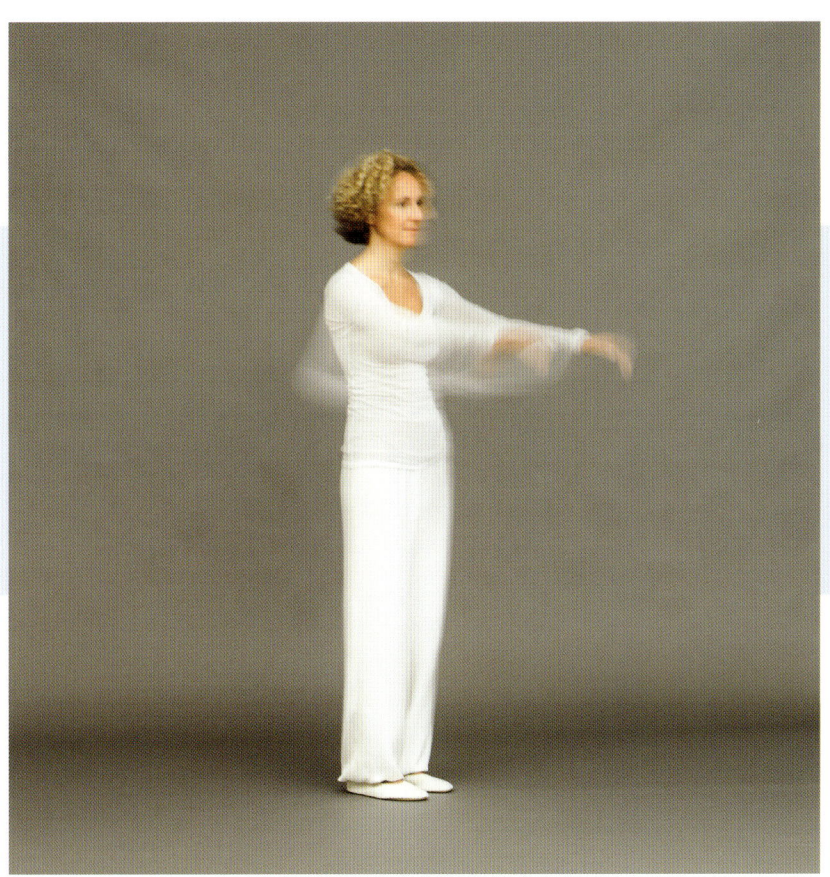
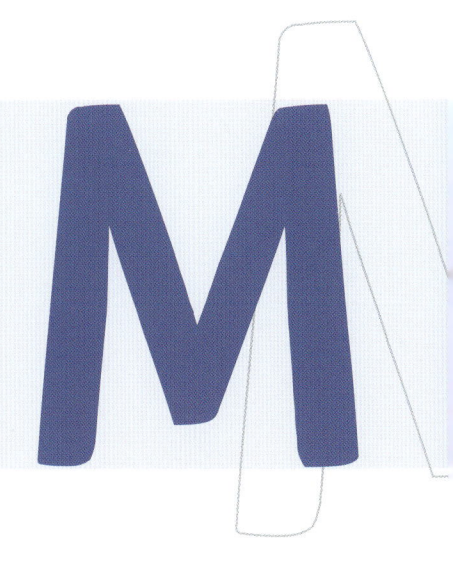

Supple sensing

- ☼ Encourages warmth, harmony, calm
- ☼ Regulates and deepens breathing
- ☼ Counteracts rigidity and hardening
- ☼ Stimulates life processes

Inner picture
Imagine your arms and legs are gliding through warm water or long, soft grass. Connect sensitively and empathetically with these surroundings.

Consonant Exercises

Arm movement I

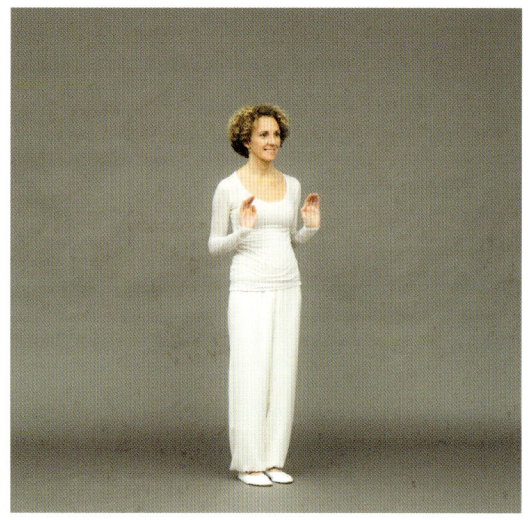

1 Stand upright. Feel a connection to the earth with your feet. Keep your knees loose and breathe calmly. Place your hands facing out at chest height. Rest your gaze on the horizon. The movement impulse will emanate from your shoulder blades.

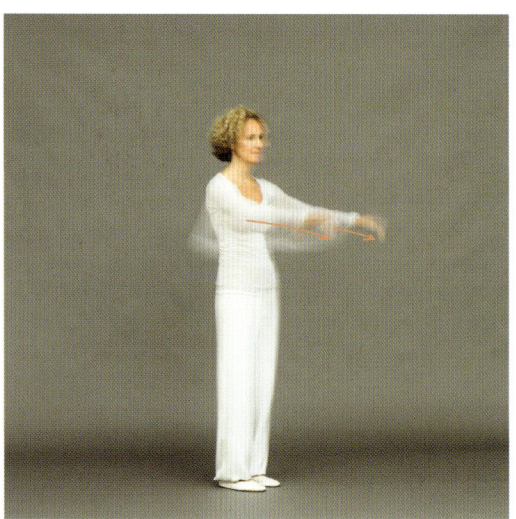

2 Move your arms gently forwards, bending your palms downwards as you go.

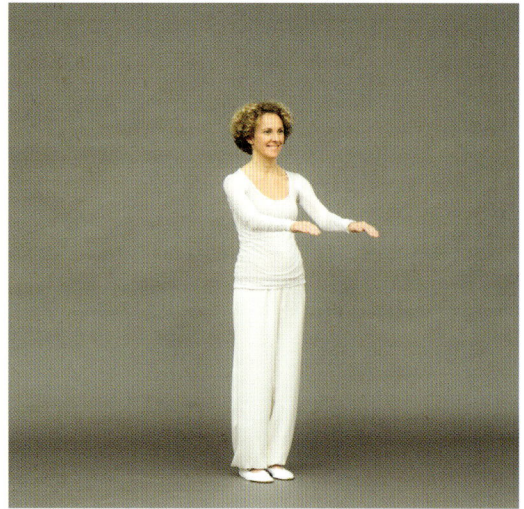

3 Pause with outstretched arms at chest height.

Consonant Exercises

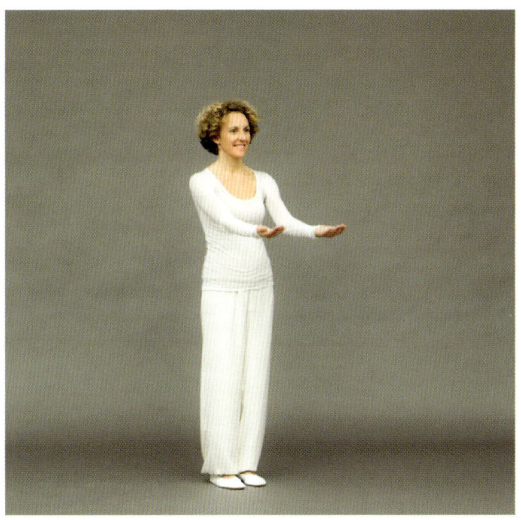

4 Turn your palms upwards.

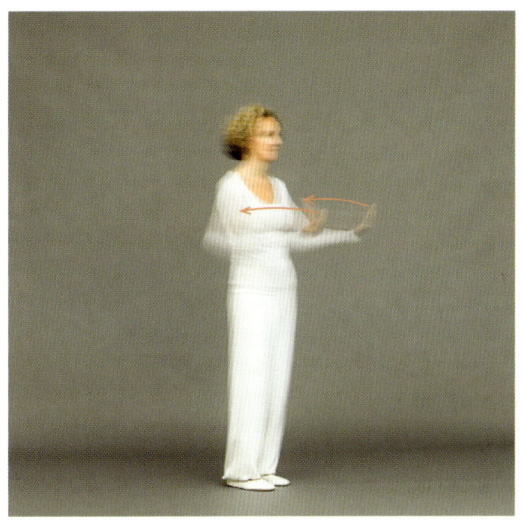

5 Pull your arms back towards your body.

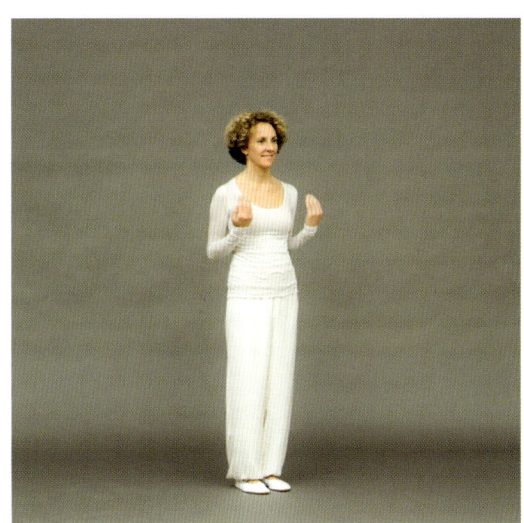

6 And release. Repeat as many times as you wish.

M

Consonant Exercises

Arm movement II

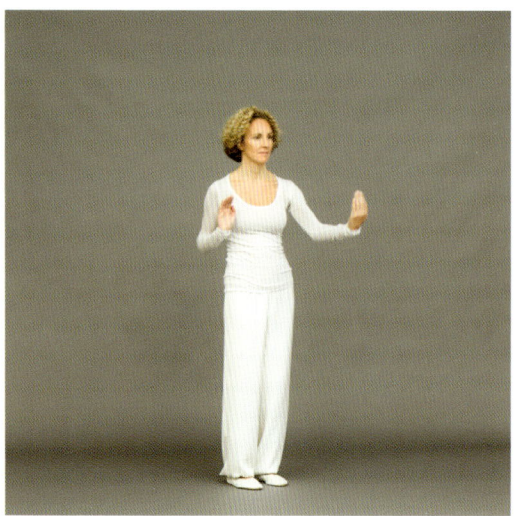 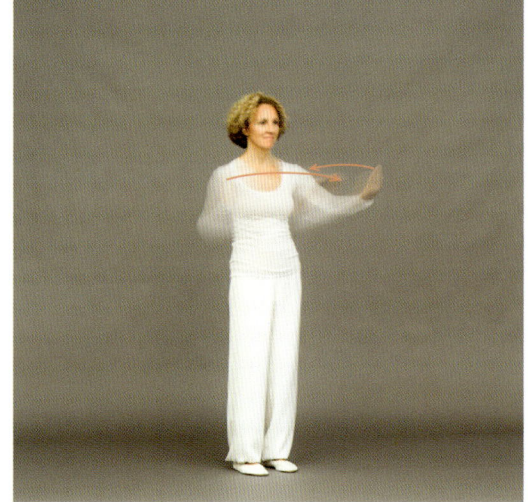

1 Stand upright. Feel a connection to the earth with your feet. Keep your knees loose and breathe calmly. Keep one hand as you did in 'Arm movement I' on page 108, and push out the other with your palm facing inwards. Rest your gaze on the horizon. The movement impulse will emanate from your shoulder blades.

2 Move both arms towards each other – one arm forwards, the other towards the body. Then turn both palms the opposite way and perform the contrary motion. Repeat as many times as you like.

Consonant Exercises

Arm movement III

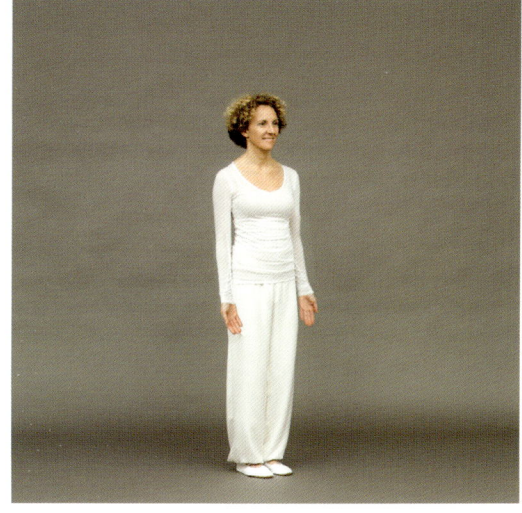

1 Stand upright. Feel a connection to the earth with your feet. Keep your knees loose and breathe calmly. Place your arms by your sides with palms facing to the front. Rest your gaze on the horizon. The movement impulse will emanate from your shoulder blades.

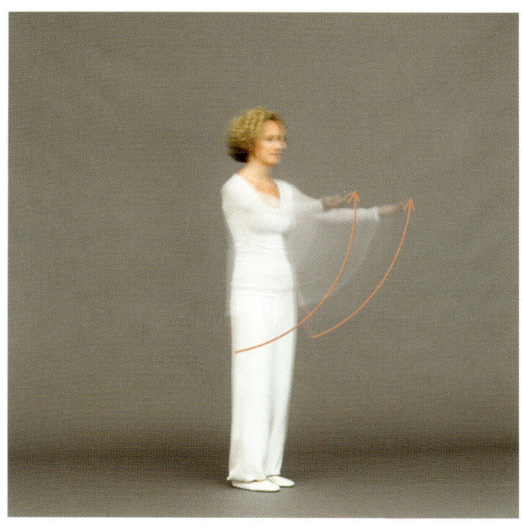

2 Sweep your arms upwards to shoulder height.

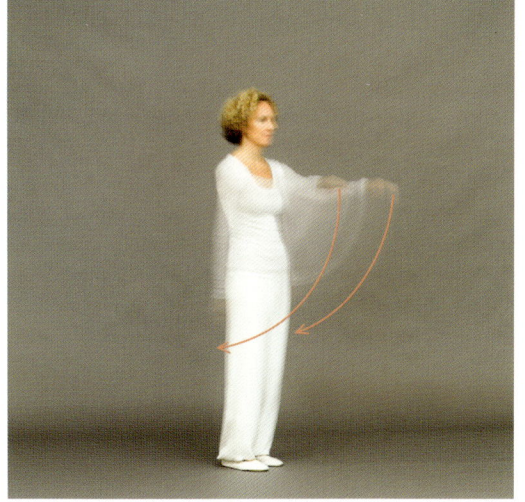

3 Now turn your palms down and sweep your arms back down to your sides. Repeat as many times as you wish.

Consonant Exercises

Arm movement IV

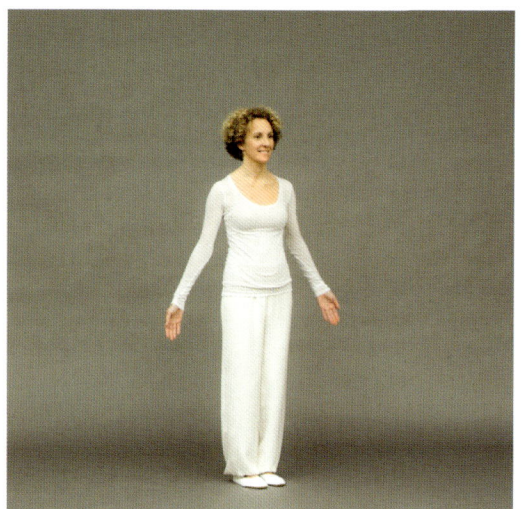 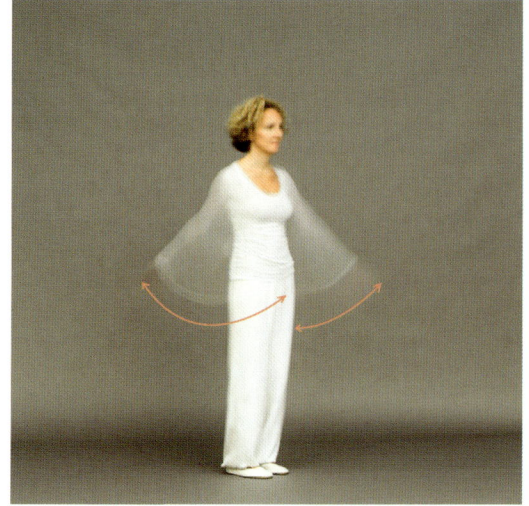

1 Stand upright. Feel a connection to the earth with your feet. Keep your knees loose and breathe calmly. Place your arms low, slightly away from your body, with palms facing to the front. Rest your gaze on the horizon. The movement impulse will emanate from your shoulder blades.

2 Sweep your arms forwards in front of you. Then turn your palms to face behind you and move your arms back again to the starting position. Repeat as many times as you like.

Consonant Exercises

Arm movement V

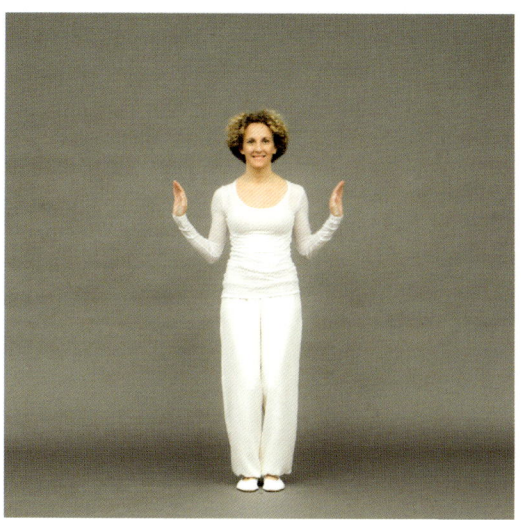

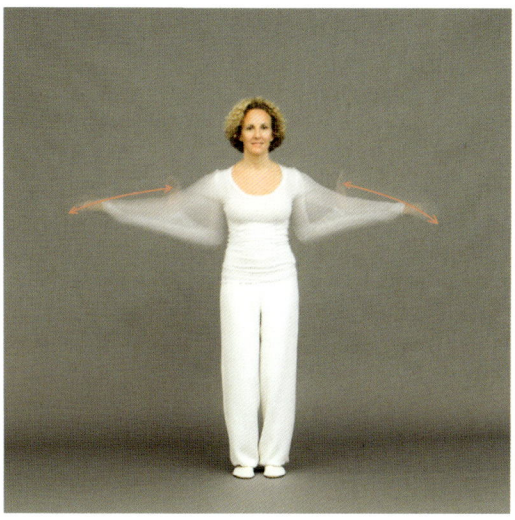

1 Stand upright. Feel a connection to the earth with your feet. Keep your knees loose and breathe calmly. Place your hands either side of your shoulders, with palms facing to each side. Rest your gaze on the horizon. The movement impulse will emanate from your shoulder blades.

2 Gently push your arms out sideways. Then turn your palms towards your body and lead them back again. Repeat as many times as you like.

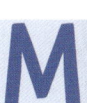

Consonant Exercises

Arm movement VI

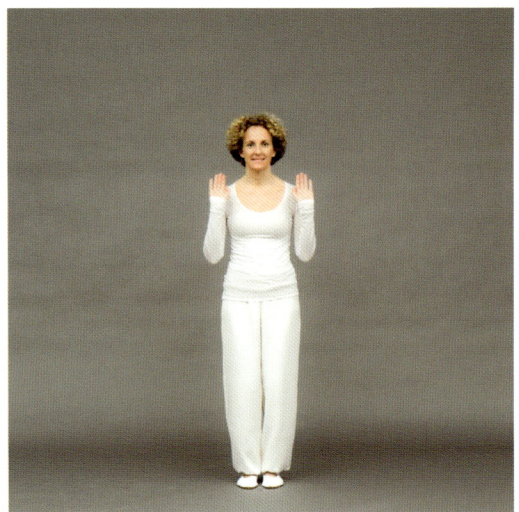 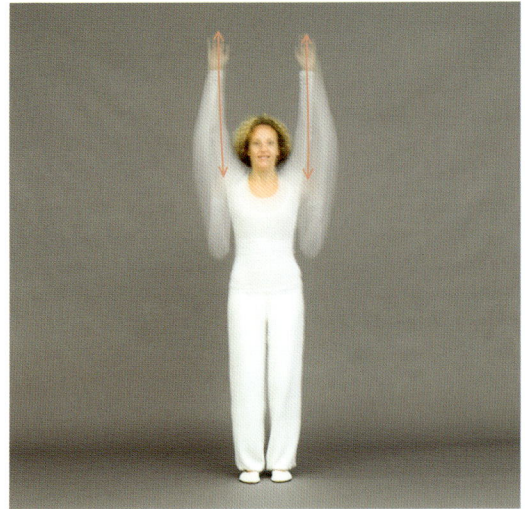

1 Stand upright. Feel a connection to the earth with your feet. Keep your knees loose and breathe calmly. Place your hands up by your shoulders, palms facing out in front of you. Rest your gaze on the horizon. The movement impulse will emanate from your shoulder blades.

2 Reach your arms upwards and draw them back again. Repeat as many times as you like.

Consonant Exercises

Leg movement I

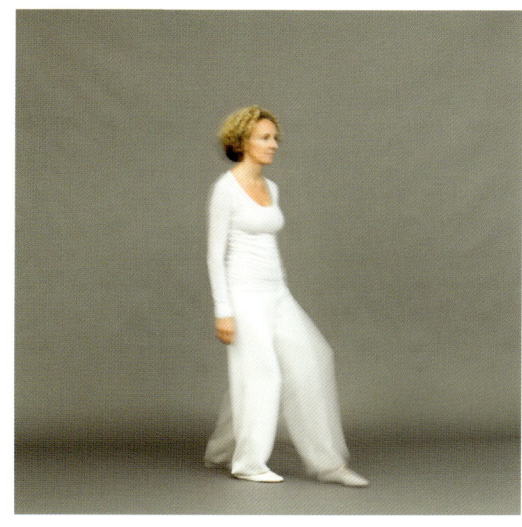

1 With your arms by your side, step your left leg forward, toe first. Bring your right leg forward to join it and lower your left heel. Then do this movement starting with your right leg. This can be done backwards as well as forwards.

Combined movement I

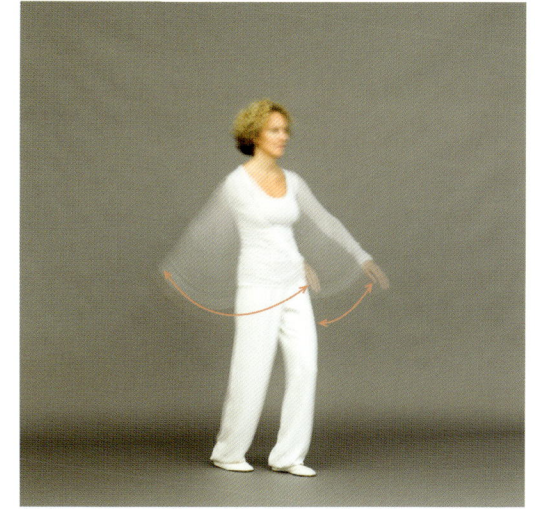

1 Sweep your arms forwards and backwards as in 'Arm movement IV', and accompany their forward and backward movement with a swaying, rocking step. As you do this, shift your weight alternately to the front and back foot, and each time you rock forwards take a step forwards also.

Combined movement II

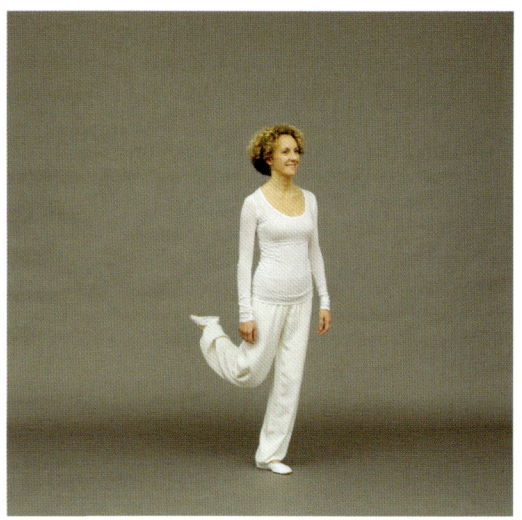 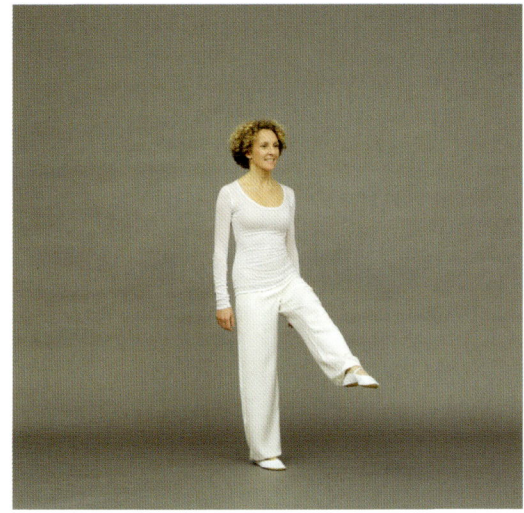

1 With your arms by your sides, bend your right leg back behind you. Then, with a swift kicking motion, sweep your right knee into the back of your left knee and kick your left leg out.

2 Land on your right foot with your left leg stretched out. Repeat the action with your left leg first.

Consonant Exercises

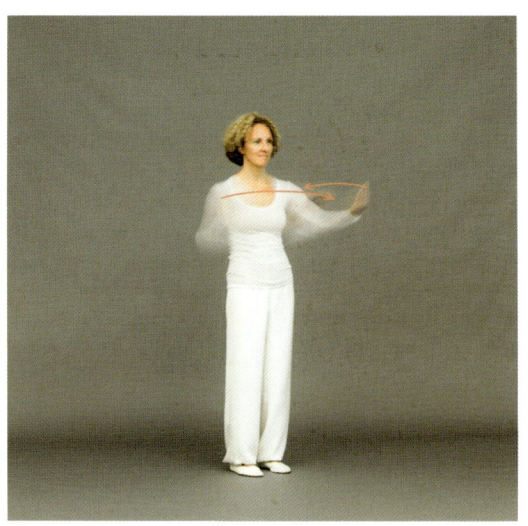 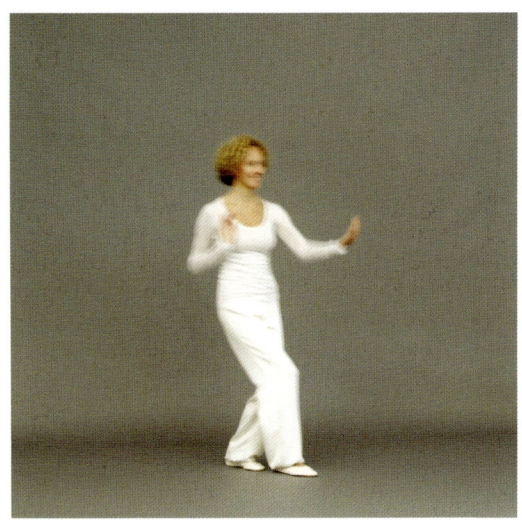

3 As you did in 'Arm movement II', move both arms in opposing directions, turn and repeat.

4 Add the leg-kicking movement at the same time and repeat.

Tip
☼ Try to perform the movement slowly and smoothly.

Consonant Exercises

Combined movement III

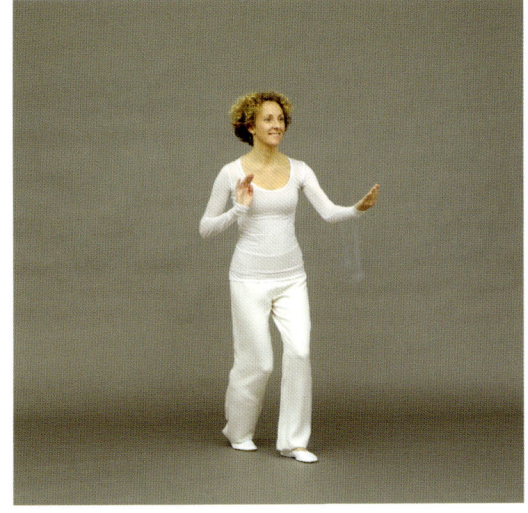

1 This movement is an extended version of 'Combined movement II' on page 116.

Consonant Exercises

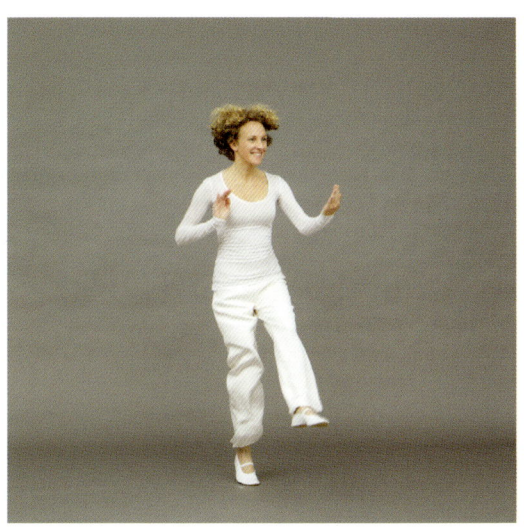

2 Add energy to the movement by taking a little leap as you sweep your bent knee forwards and kick your straight leg out.

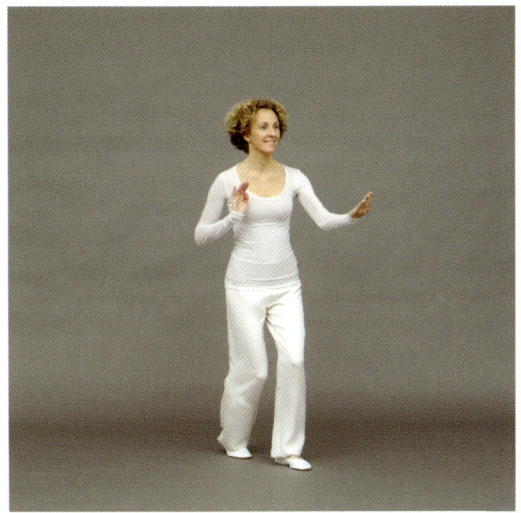

3 These can also be done as backwards jumps, with the outstretched front leg sweeping back to cause the opposite leg to bend out behind you.

Tips

- Take a little step between leaps to keep moving.
- Two or four 'knee kicks' correspond to one slow arm movement.
- Repeat this movement as many times as you like.
- Keep your inner picture in mind and feel its resistance.
- Allow the consonant to work within you for a while after you finish.

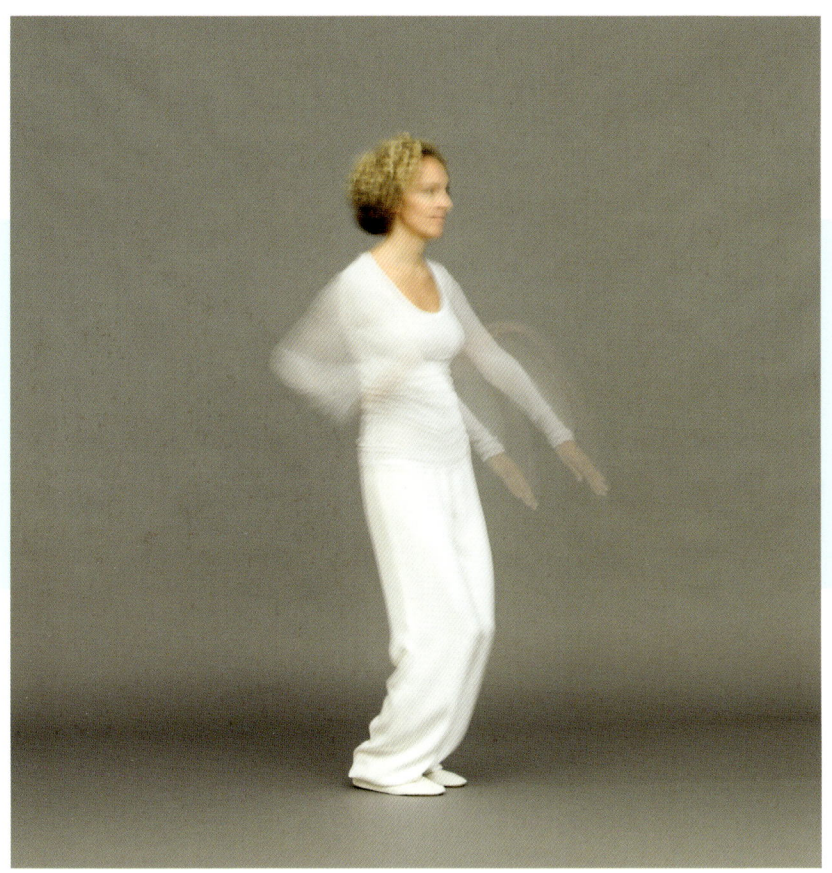 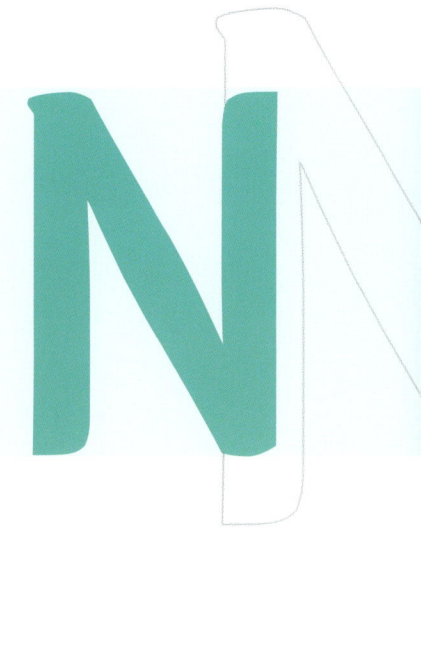

Quickly withdrawing

- ✺ Encourages sensitivity, structure, interest in surroundings
- ✺ Draws us into ourselves
- ✺ Helps soothe digestive problems

Inner picture
Imagine you are absorbing the impression of unfamiliar natural surroundings. Attend sensitively to something in your vicinity, before quickly and dynamically withdrawing from it again.

Consonant Exercises

Arm movement

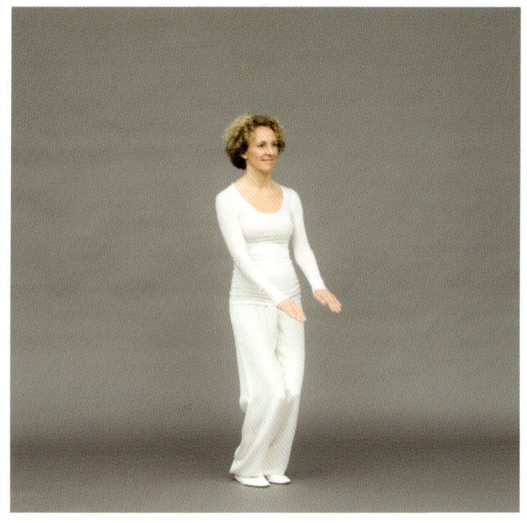

1 Stand upright. Feel a connection to the earth with your feet. Keep your knees loose and breathe calmly. Extend your arms downwards in front of you, with palms facing down. Rest your gaze on the horizon. The movement impulse will emanate from your shoulder blades.

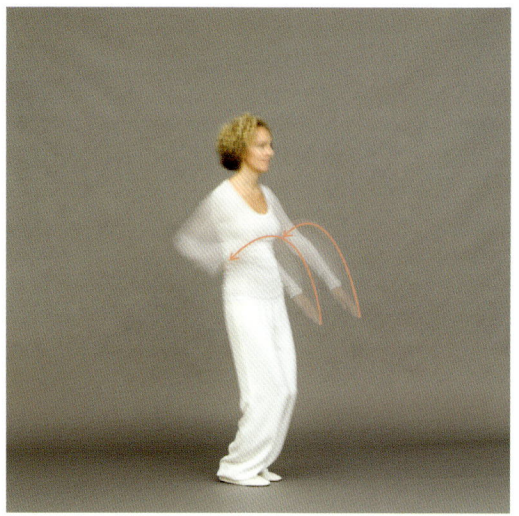

2 Move your hands back towards your body in a withdrawing gesture. Feel free to add a bend in your knees to exaggerate the withdrawing gesture.

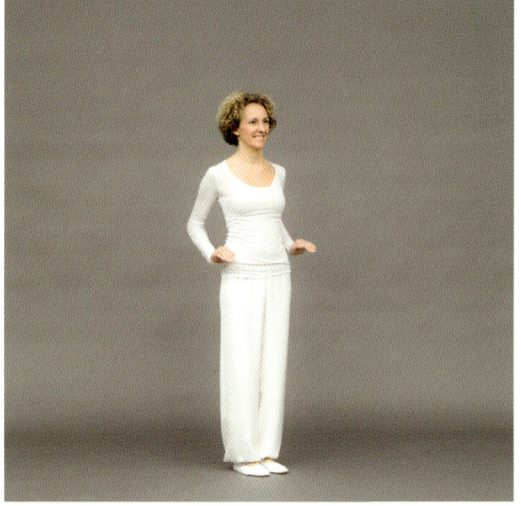

3 Draw your hands up to hip level, palms facing down.

Leg movement

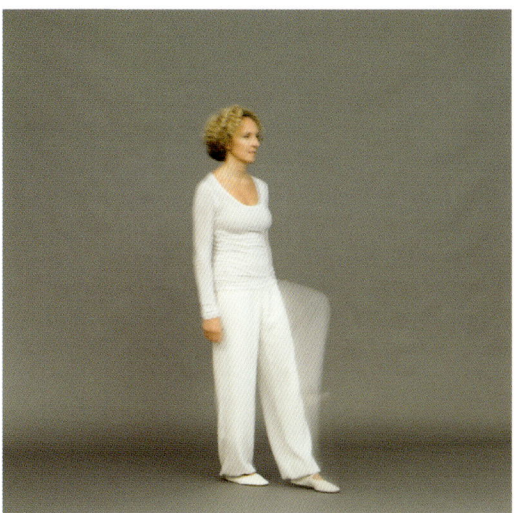

1 Touch the ground with your left toe and then let the leg spring back upwards again.

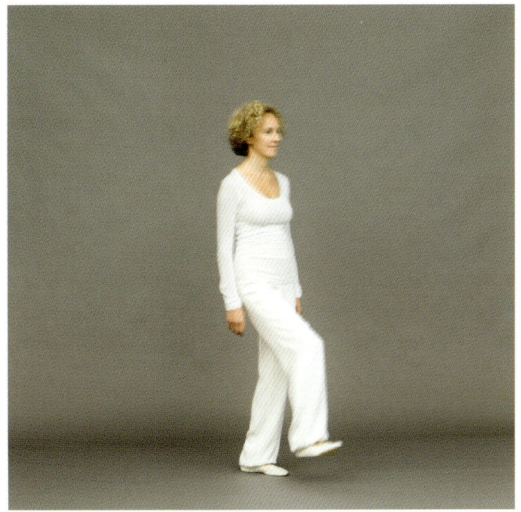

2 Repeat this with your right leg.

Combined movement

As you move your arms, either add the toe withdrawal movement too or jump gently forwards or backwards.

Tips

- Repeat this movement as many times as you like.
- Keep your inner picture in mind and move within it.
- Allow the consonant to work within you for a while after you finish.

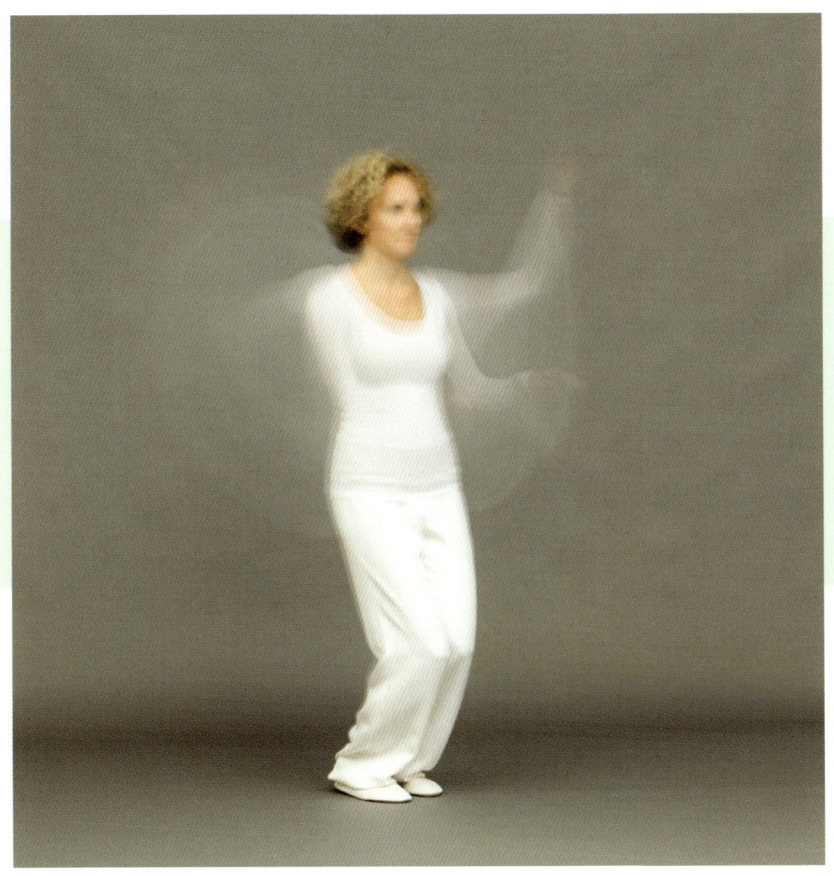
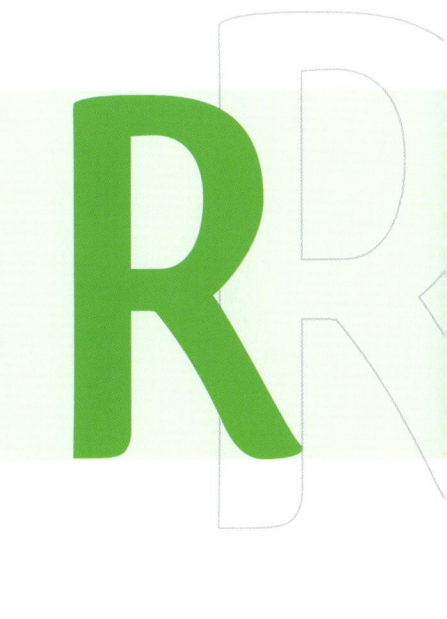

Revolving

- Encourages flexibility, liveliness, stimulation
- Regulates and strengthens breathing
- Brings movement to rigidity

Inner picture Imagine gently pulling over, in a car or on a bike, on a country road to admire a beautiful view. Your limbs move but your head remains still, mesmerised.

Consonant Exercises

Arm movement

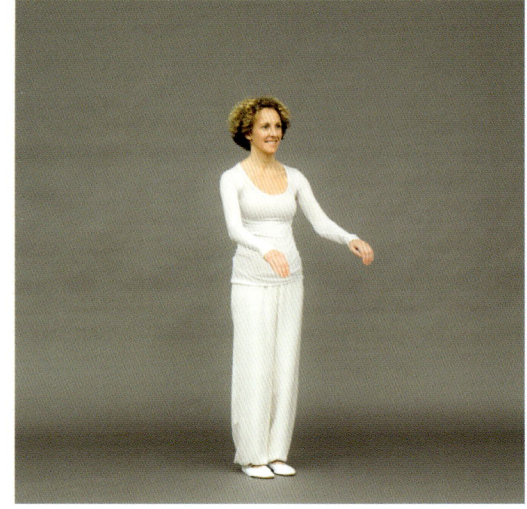

1 Stand upright. Feel a connection to the earth with your feet. Keep your knees loose and breathe calmly. Extend your arms out level with your hips, with palms facing down. Rest your gaze on the horizon. The movement impulse will emanate from your shoulder blades.

Consonant Exercises

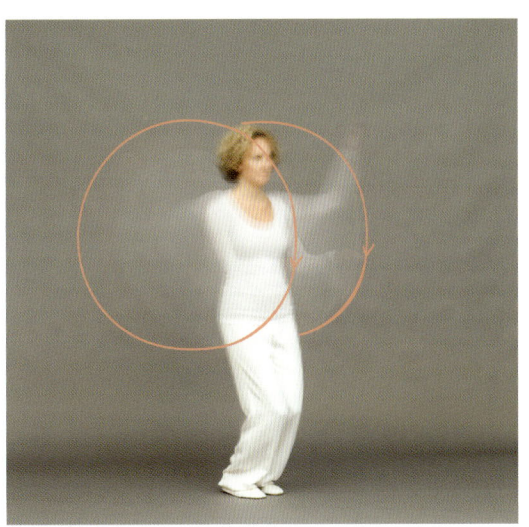 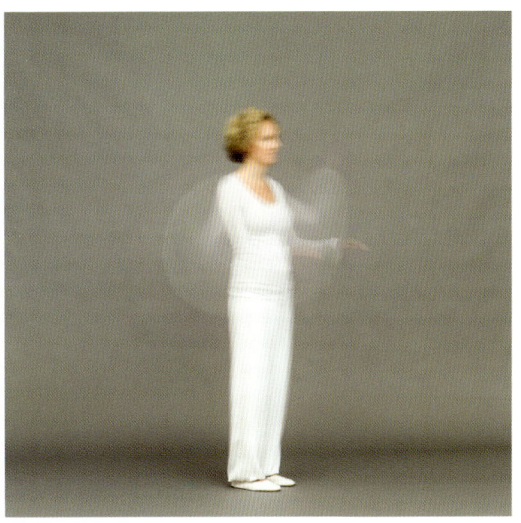

2 With elbows slightly bent, rotate your arms in wide circles from behind you to the front. If you wish, you can gently bend your knees as you go.

3 After a few revolutions, stand up straight again in a neutral position.

R

Consonant Exercises

Leg movement

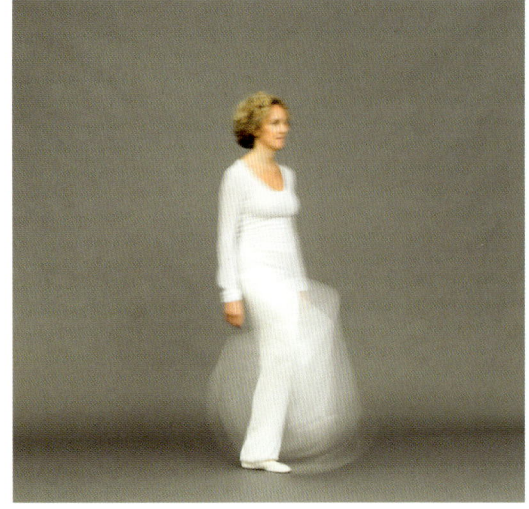

1 Echo the shape of the 'Arm movement' on page 126-127 by revolving one leg at a time. Alternate your leg after each revolution.

Consonant Exercises

Combined movement

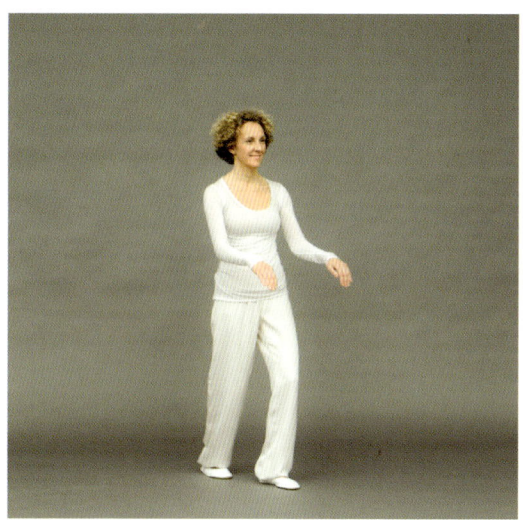

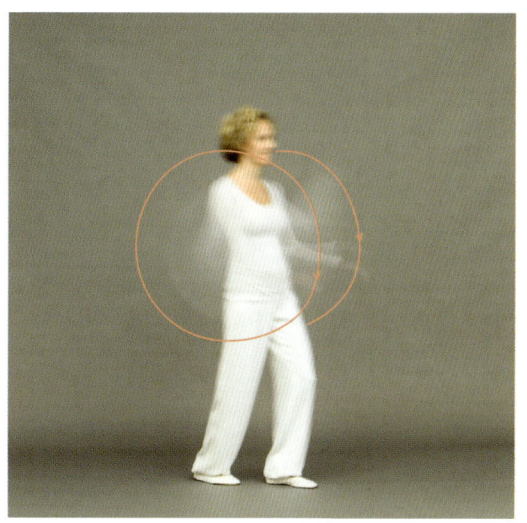

1 Stand upright. Feel a connection to the earth with your feet. Keep your knees loose and breathe calmly. Hold your arms level with your stomach, with palms facing down. Rest your gaze on the horizon. The movement impulse will emanate from your shoulder blades.

2 Revolve your arms as before, bending and stretching your knees in a stepping motion as you do so. The arm movement can be performed in wider or tighter circles depending on your preference.

Tips

✧ Repeat this movement as many times as you like.

✧ Keep your inner picture in mind and move within it.

✧ Allow the consonant to work within you for a while after you finish.

R

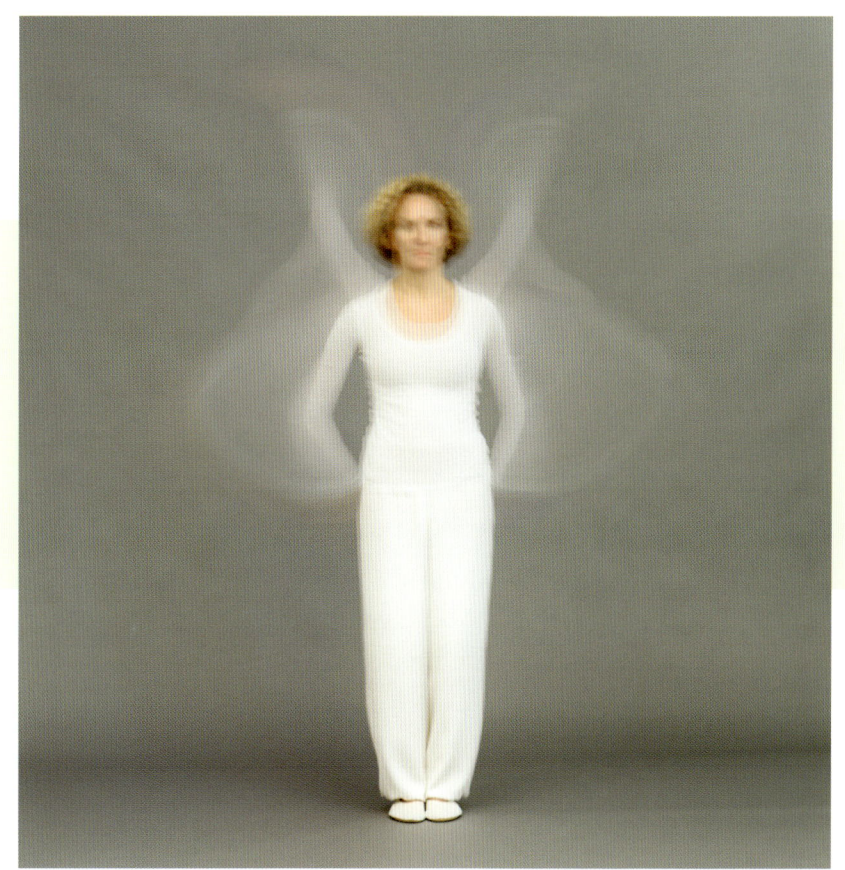
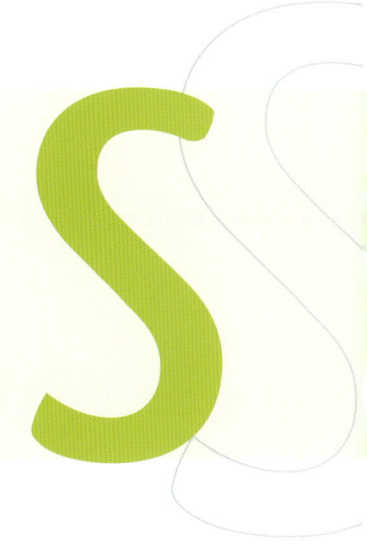

Enlivening and formative

- Encourages strength, transformation, warmth
- Brings structure and calm
- Balances polar processes

Inner picture Imagine two contrary streams working together: a rising one, bringing dynamic springtime forces of birth and vitality; and a descending one, bringing maturation, density and substance. This contrary movement resembles nature's processes of growth and decay throughout the year.

Consonant Exercises

Arm movement I

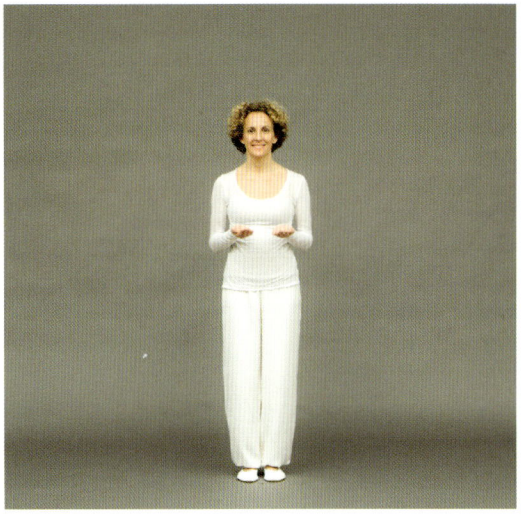

1 Stand upright. Feel a connection to the earth with your feet. Keep your knees loose and breathe calmly. Hold your hands out in front of you, palms facing up. Rest your gaze on the horizon. The movement impulse will emanate from your shoulder blades.

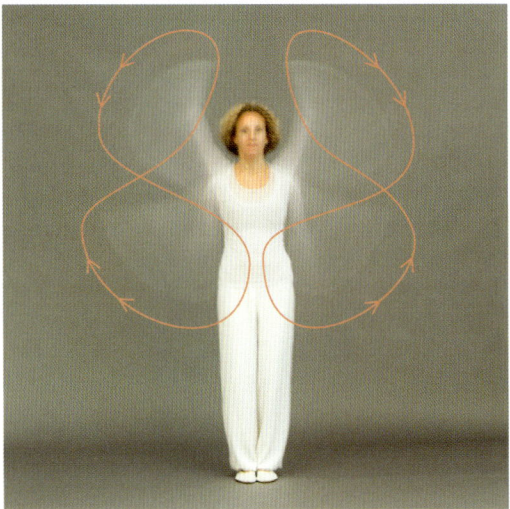

2 With both arms mirroring each other, draw a figure of eight in front of you. Start outward and upward above your head and then swoop in through the whole figure.

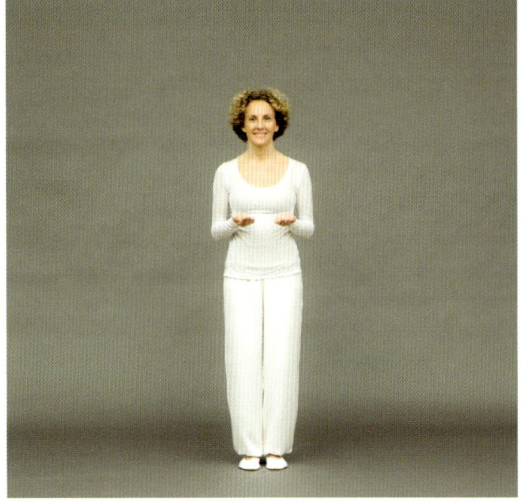

3 Release your hands back to the starting position.

Consonant Exercises

Arm movement II

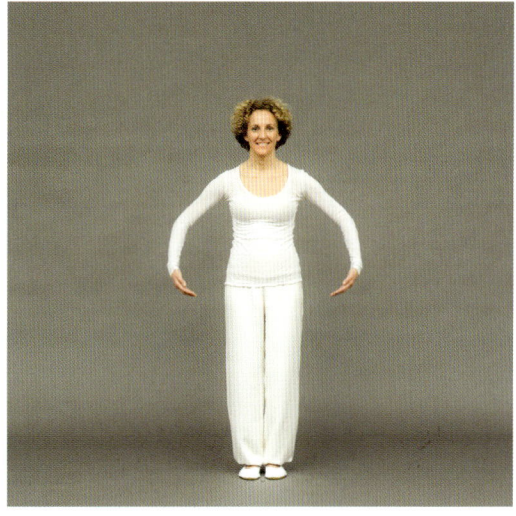

1 Stand upright. Feel a connection to the earth with your feet. Keep your knees loose and breathe calmly. Hold your arms wide and low as if you are carrying a big beach ball. Rest your gaze on the horizon. The movement impulse will emanate from your shoulder blades.

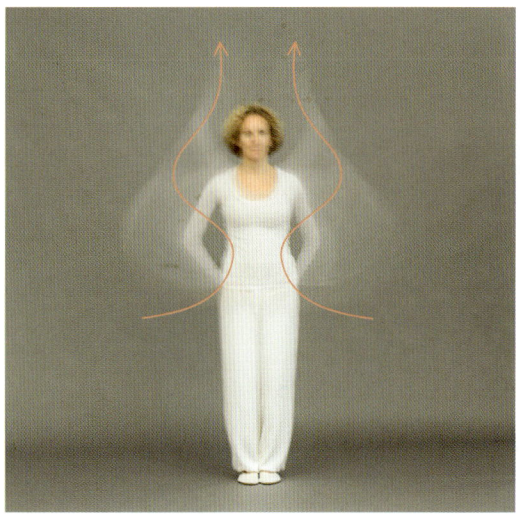

2 With both arms mirroring each other, make a vertical S-shape that swoops from below upwards. Start the movement by moving in towards the centre of your body before moving outwards.

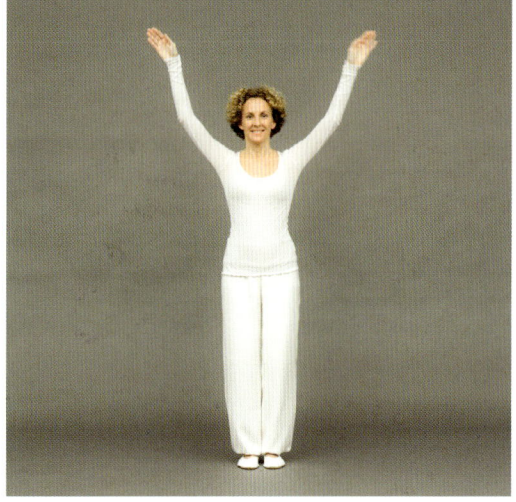

3 Let the S finish with your arms raised high and wide.

Consonant Exercises

Arm movement III

Tip

☼ This process can be done with just one arm at a time, to remedy a loss of balance.

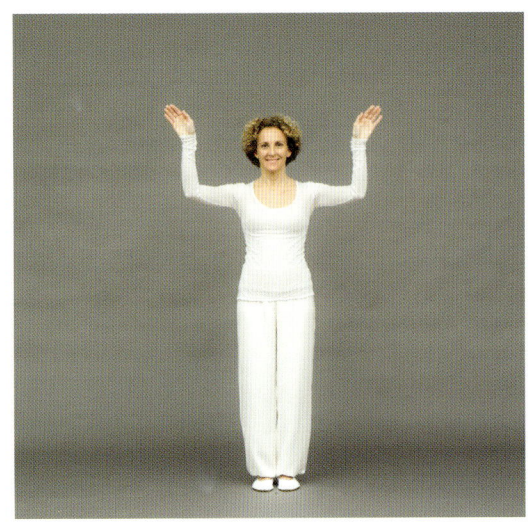

1 Stand upright. Feel a connection to the earth with your feet. Keep your knees loose and breathe calmly. Hold your hands either side of your head, palms facing forward. Rest your gaze on the horizon. The movement impulse will emanate from your shoulder blades.

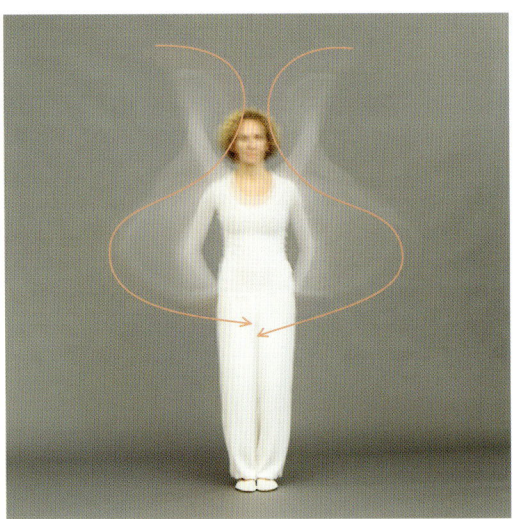

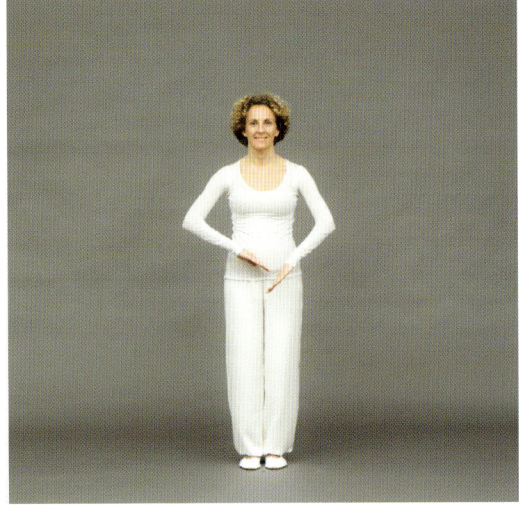

2 With both arms mirroring each other, draw a vertical S from the top down, first moving inwards, then outwards.

3 Let your arms come to rest in front of your hips.

Consonant Exercises

Leg movement I

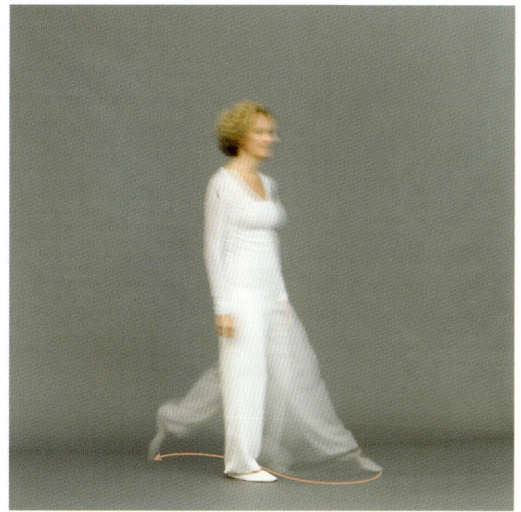

1 With your left leg, make an S shape from front to back. Take a step, then repeat with your right leg. Keep walking forwards through these S shapes.

S

Consonant Exercises

Combined movement

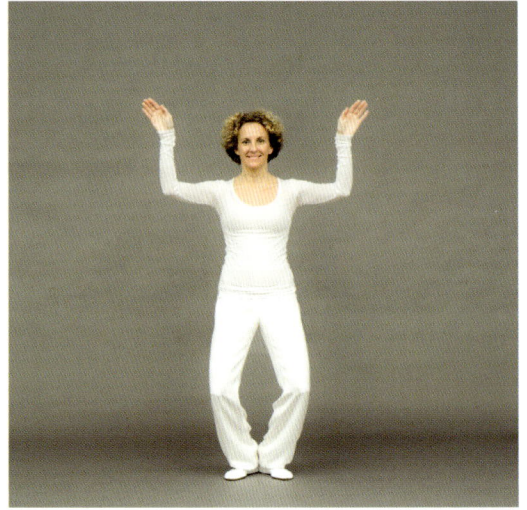

1 Stand with your legs slightly bowed. Feel a connection to the earth with your feet. Keep your knees loose and breathe calmly. Hold your hands out either side of your head as in 'Arm movement III'. Rest your gaze on the horizon. The movement impulse will emanate from your shoulder blades.

Consonant Exercises

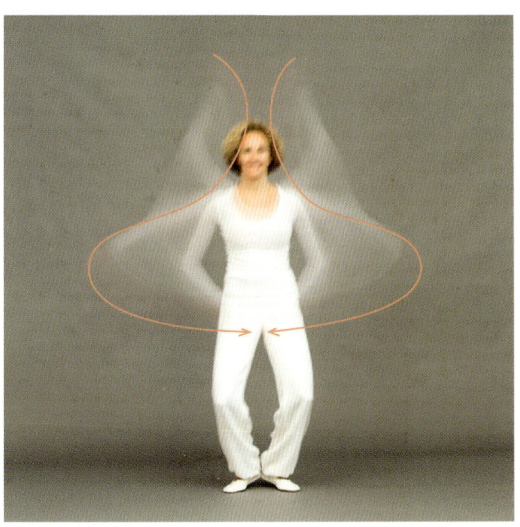 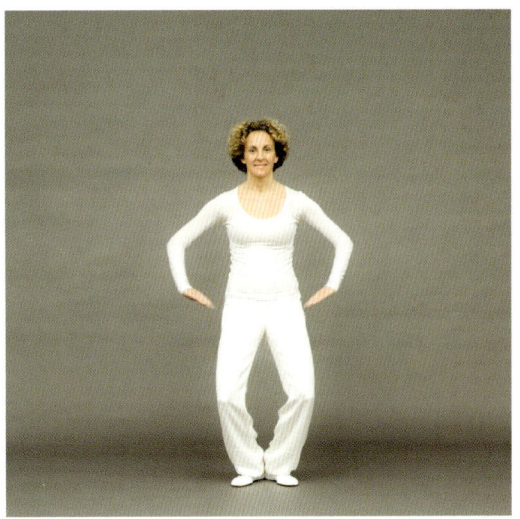

2 With both hands make an S shape from the top down. At the same time, keeping your legs in their O shape, try a small jump.

3 End with your elbows out and your hands pointing in at your hips.

Tips

✿ This exercise can also be done with asymmetrical arm movements.

✿ Repeat this movement as many times as you like.

✿ Keep your inner picture in mind and move within it.

✿ Allow the consonant to work within you for a while after you finish.

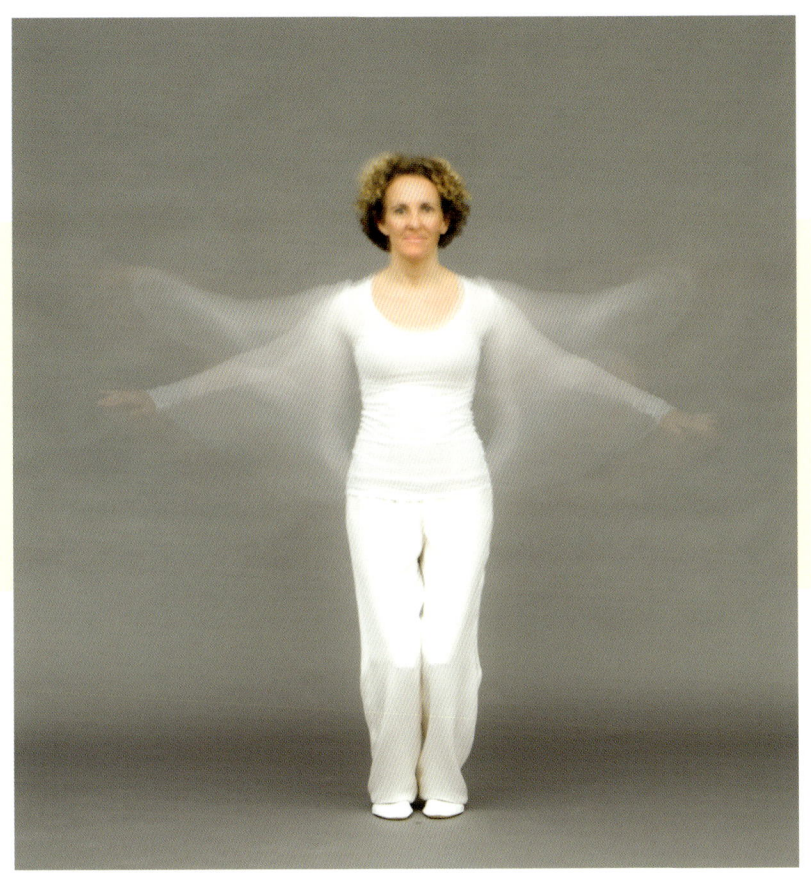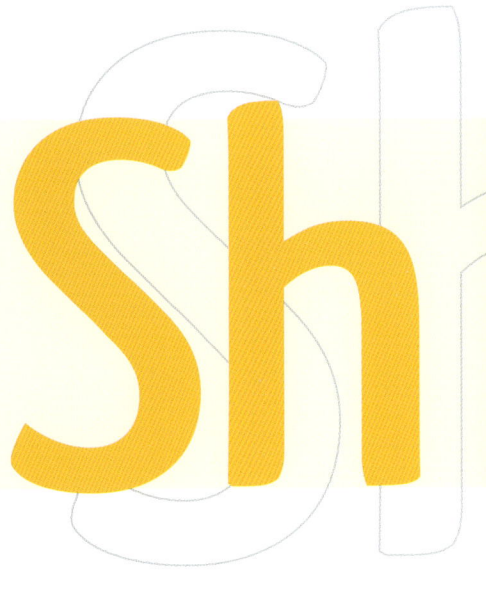

Spiralling upward

- ✺ Encourages release, relief
- ✺ Creates dynamic, internal rhythms
- ✺ Aids digestion

Inner picture Imagine mist rising from warm earth, or salt spray evaporating from a rock near the sea. The upward-moving spiral motion of the Sh gesture corresponds to energised water vapour, narrowing as it rises into the air.

Consonant Exercises

Arm movement

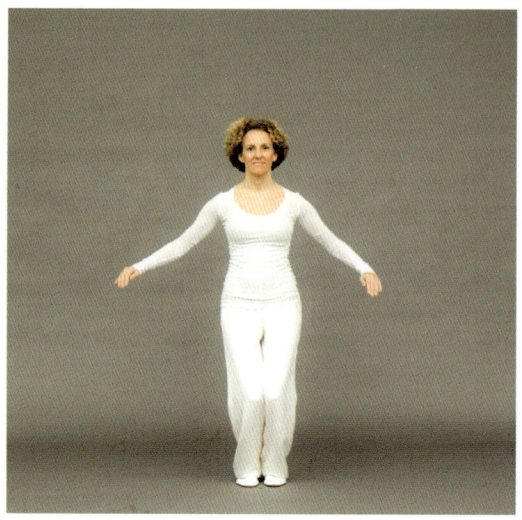

1 Stand with your knees slightly bent. Feel a connection to the earth with your feet. Keep your knees loose and breathe calmly. Hold your arms out to the sides, palms facing down. Rest your gaze on the horizon. The movement impulse will emanate from your shoulder blades.

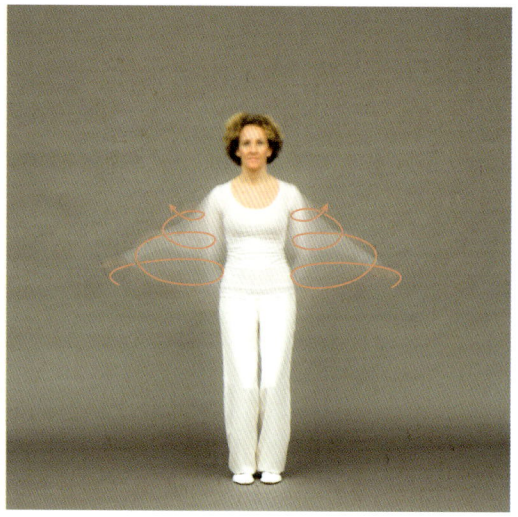

2 Spiral your arms three times, up to your shoulders, narrowing as you go higher. Your right hand should be moving clockwise and your left counterclockwise.

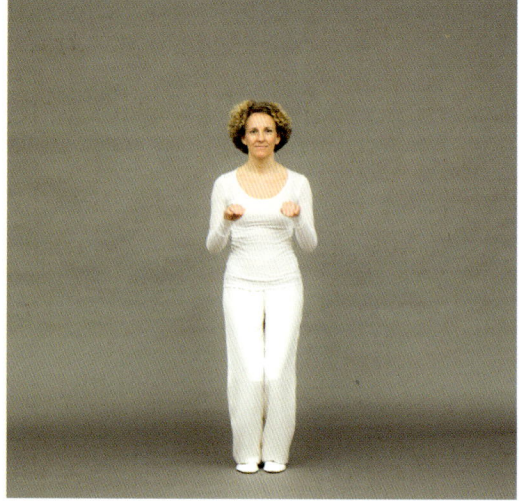

3 Bring your hands to rest level with your heart.

Consonant Exercises

Combined movement

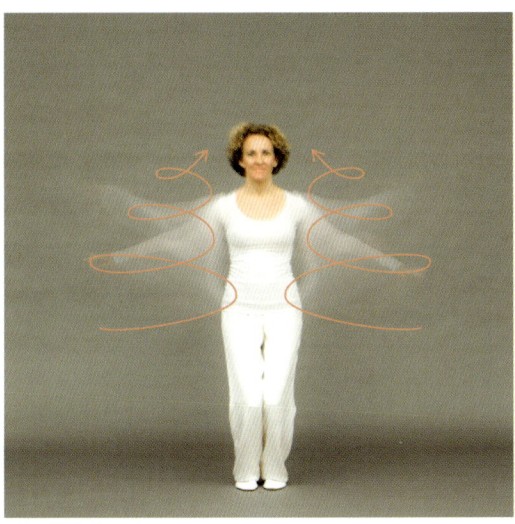 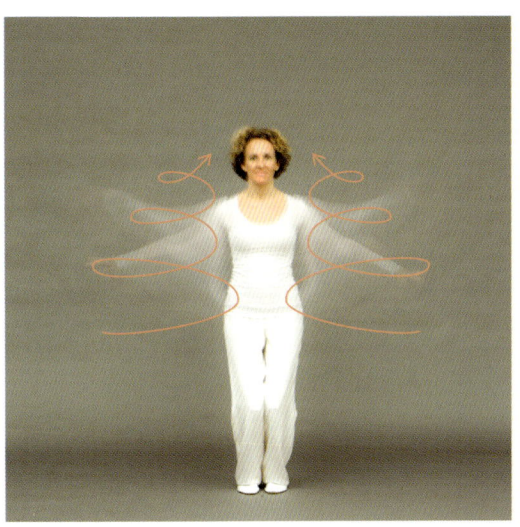

1 Accompany your spirals with rhythmic jumps or steps in the following rhythm: short, long, short (one per spiral). Then pause.

2 After a pause spiral your arms again while hopping in the rhythm: long, short, long.

Tips

- Repeat this movement as many times as you like.
- Keep your inner picture in mind and move within it.
- Allow the consonant to work within you for a while after you finish.

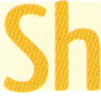

Consonant Exercises

Consonants at a Glance

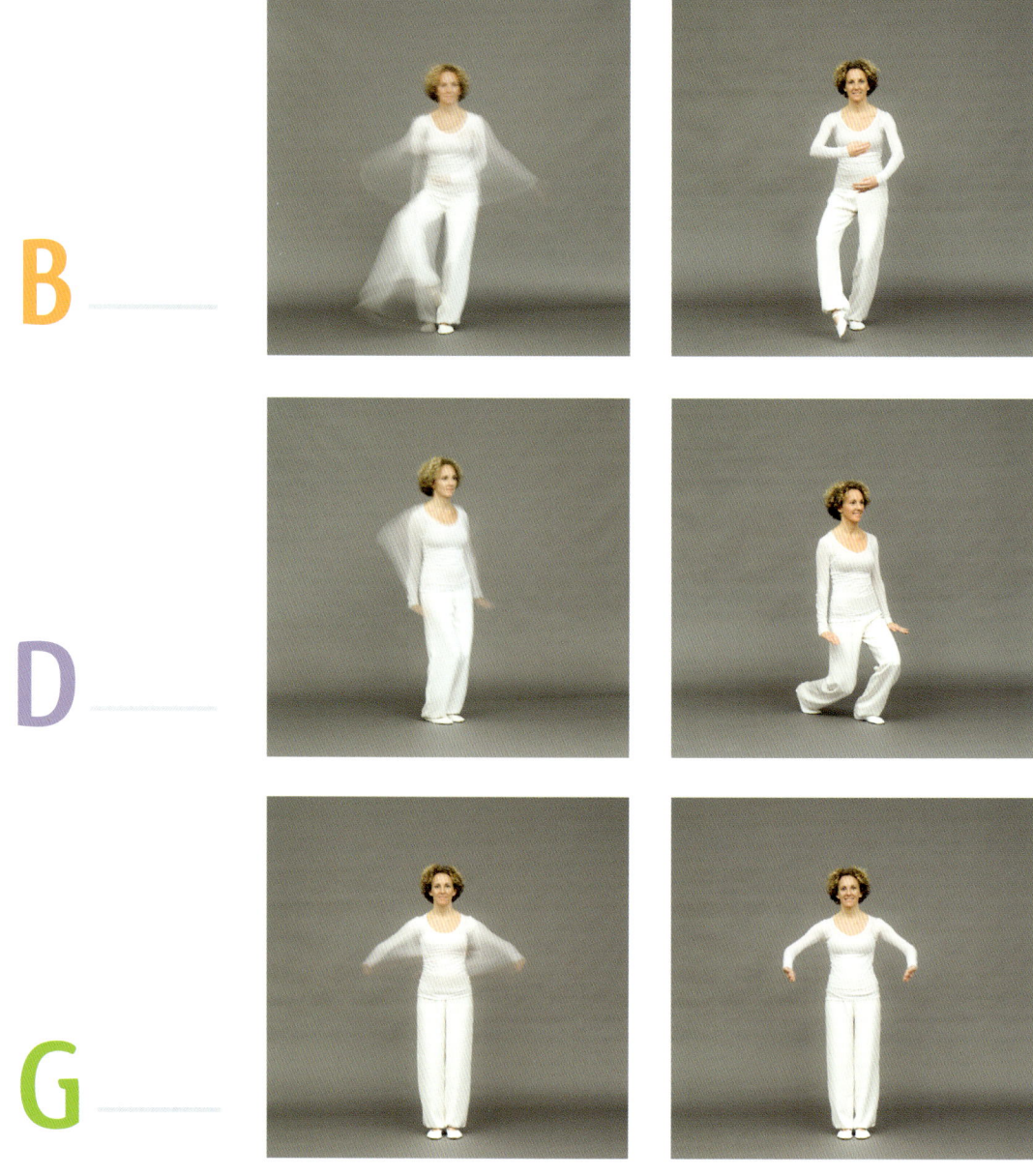

Consonant Exercises

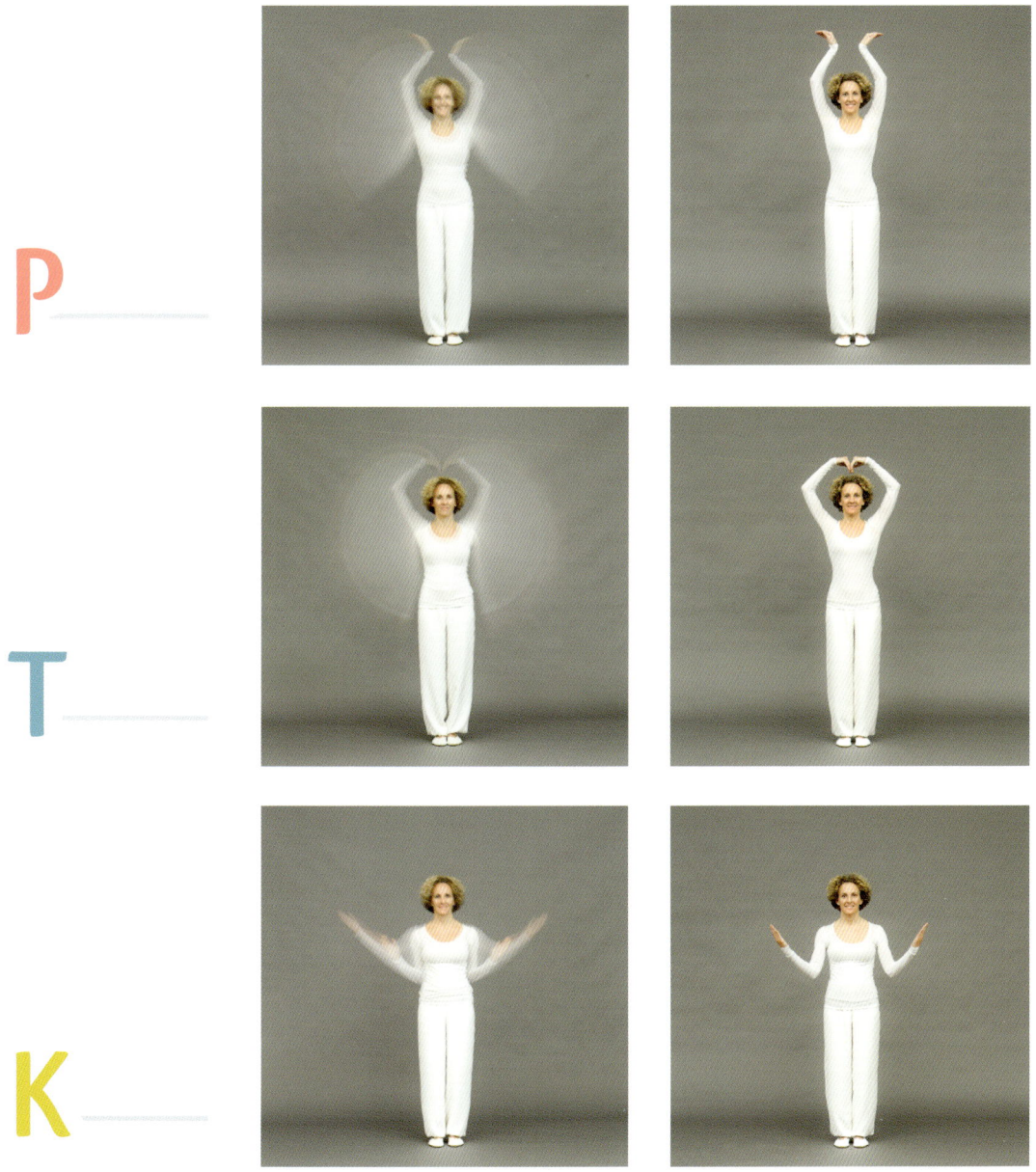

P

T

K

143

Consonant Exercises

F

L

N

S

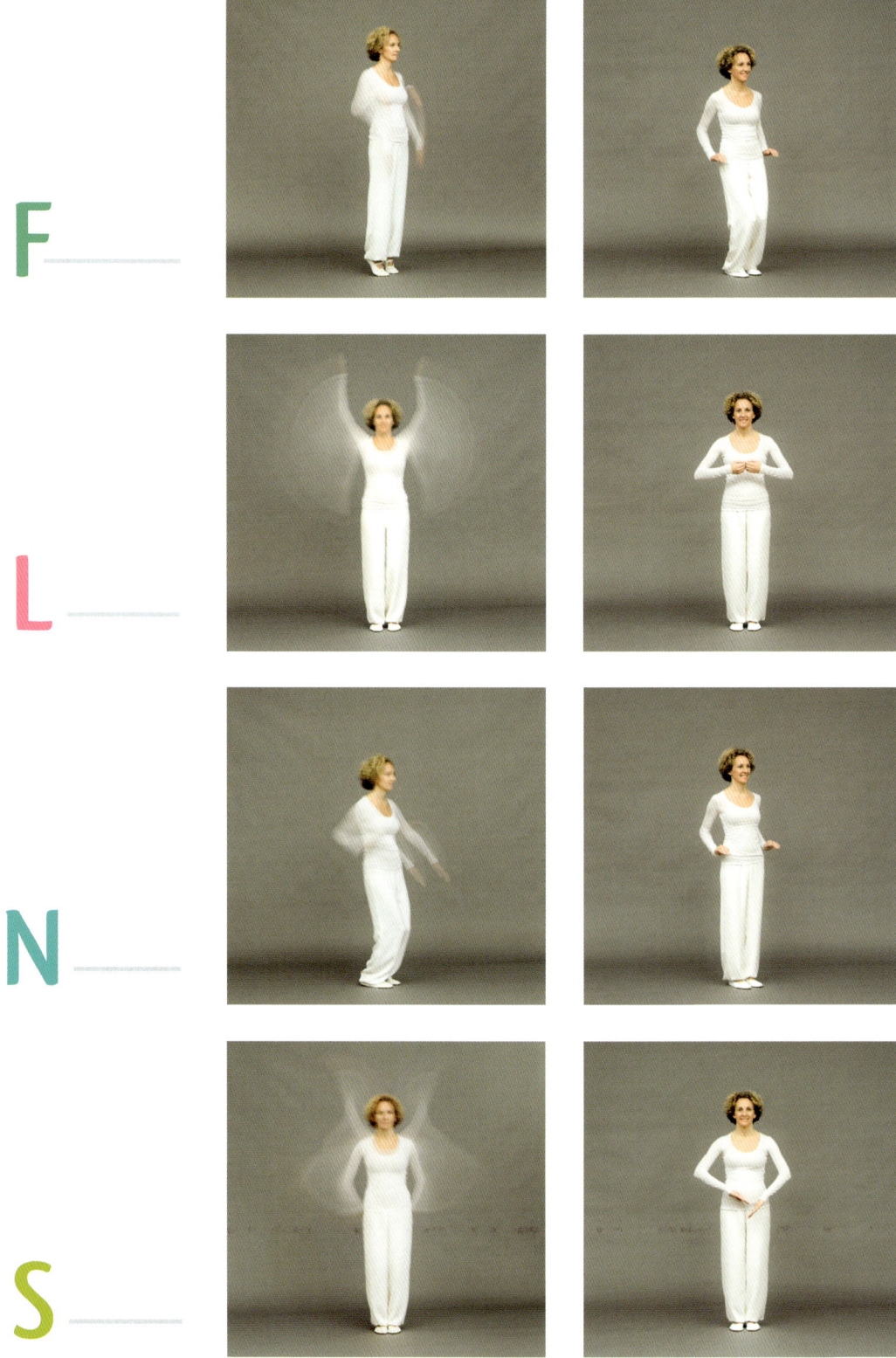

Consonant Exercises

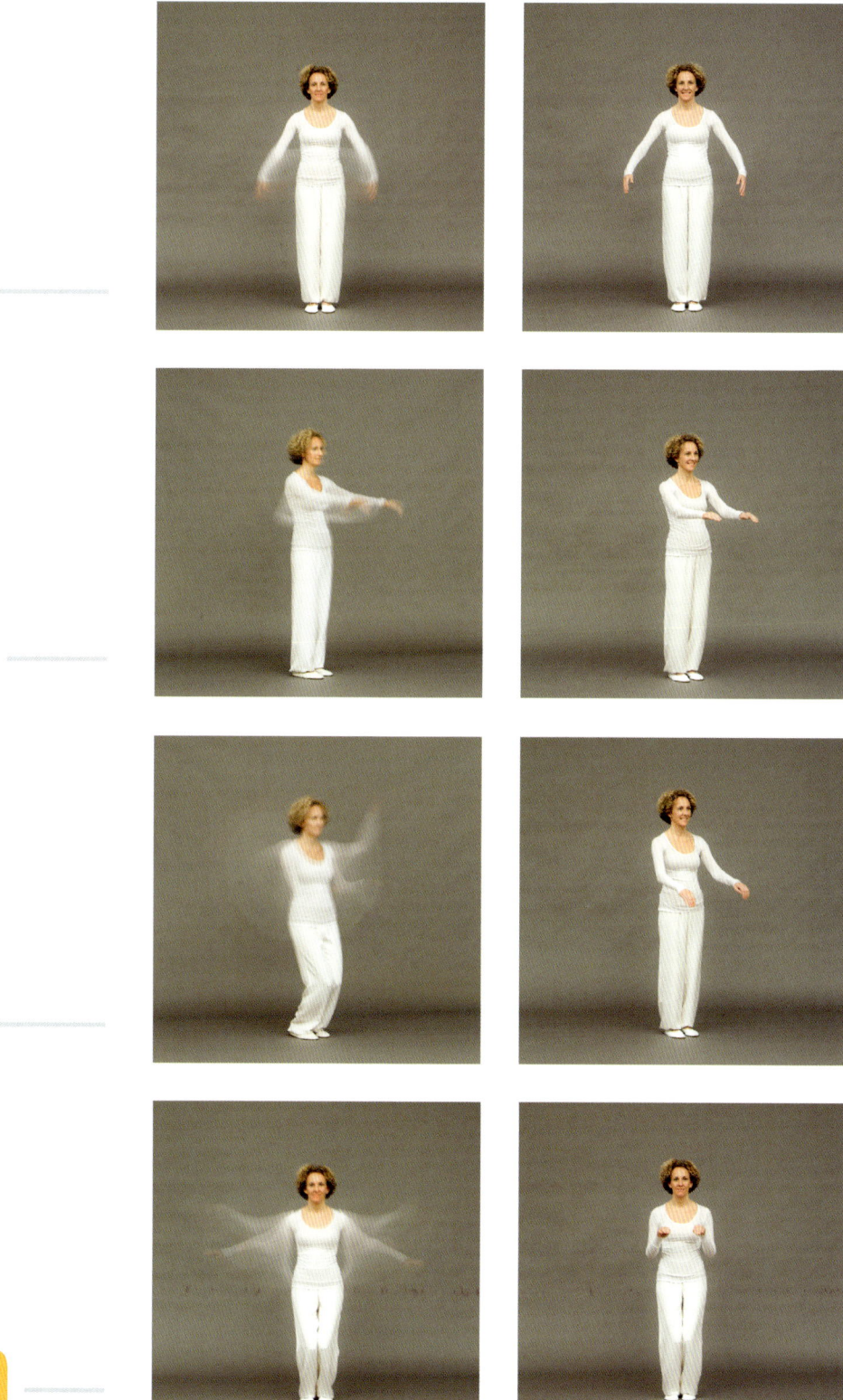

H

M

R

Sh

hope

sympathy

reverence

love

Soul Exercises

antipathy

yes

no

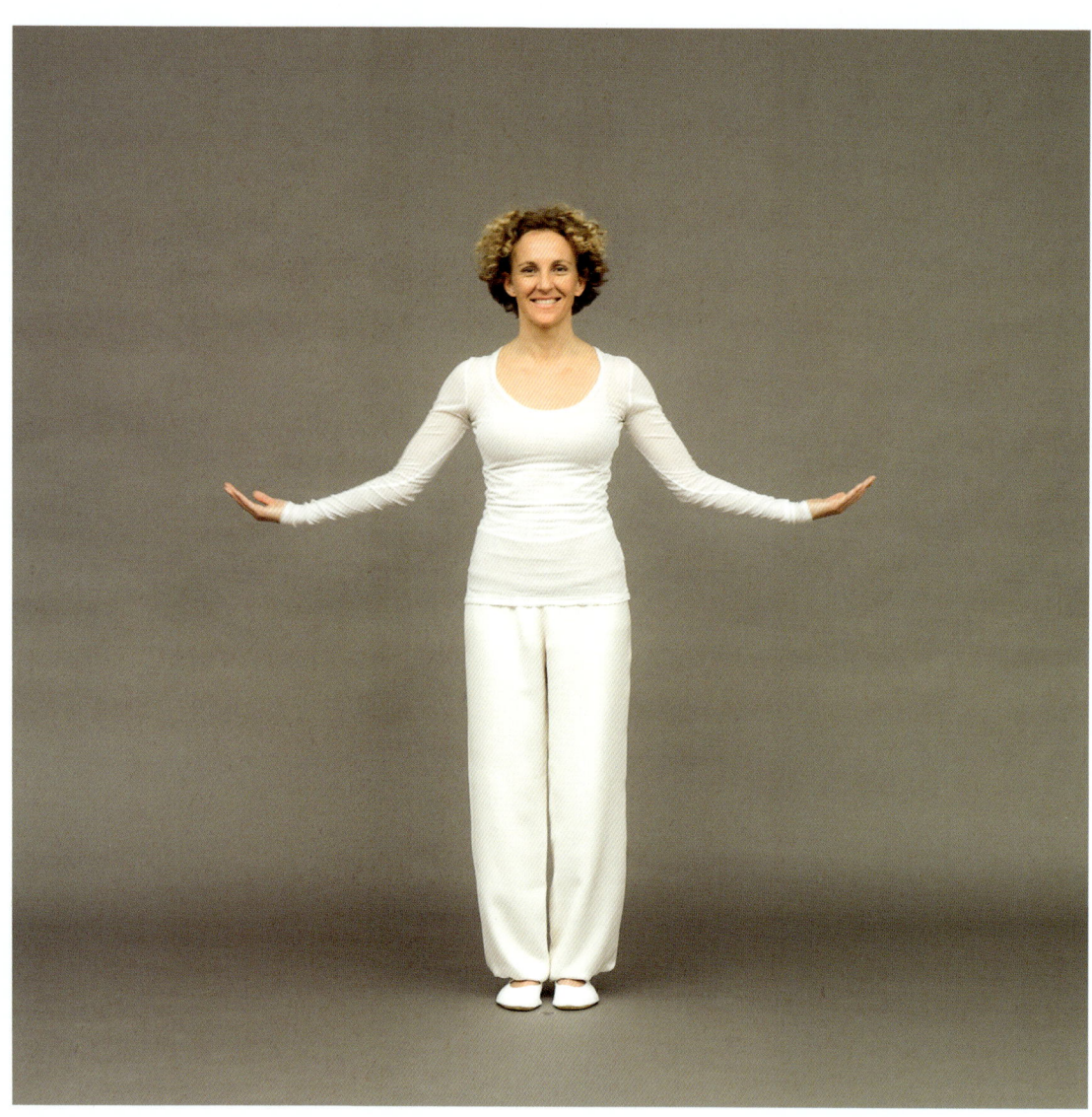

Soul Exercises

There are twelve exercises in eurythmy therapy that act on the human soul. Five of them are introduced in this section.

- ■ A (ah) Reverence
- ■ E (eh) Love
- ■ U (oo) Hope
- ■ Yes / no
- ■ Sympathy / antipathy

The connection between each of the first three vowels and their soul mood stimulates inner processes that increase our capacity for resonance. They enhance vitality and have a regulating effect on our attitude to the world around us.

The last two exercises focus on the movement of the legs or the whole human form. No eurythmy sounds are performed here.

Each of these exercises should be performed ten times in succession, if possible.

Soul Exercises

A (ah) Reverence

☼ Encourages calm, expansion, release

☼ Strengthens the immune system

☼ Helps with insomnia

Intention I release myself from all burden and reach a feeling of composure.

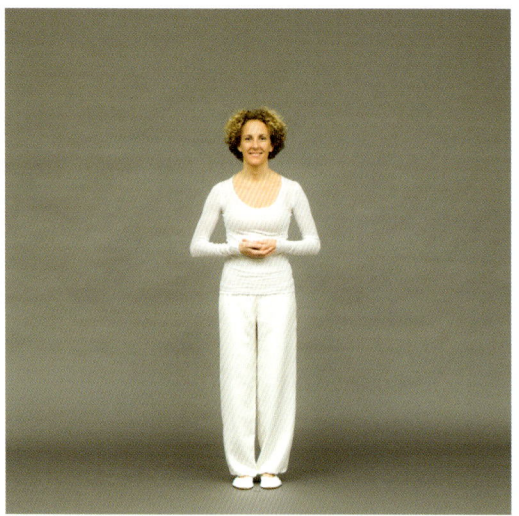 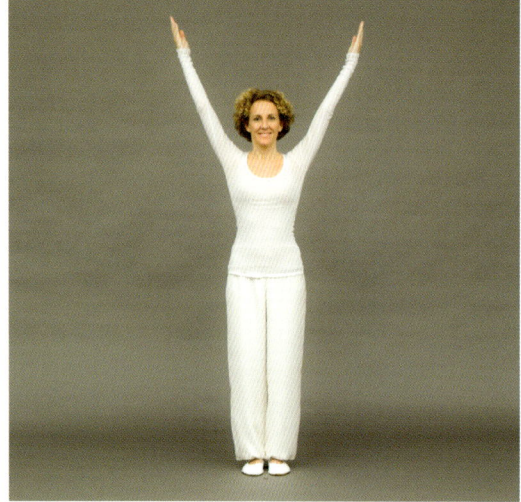

1 Stand upright. Feel a connection to the earth with your feet. Keep your knees loose and breathe calmly. Cup your hands together, level with your diaphragm. Rest your gaze on the horizon. The movement impulse will emanate from your heart.

2 Stretch your arms upwards at an angle.

Soul Exercises

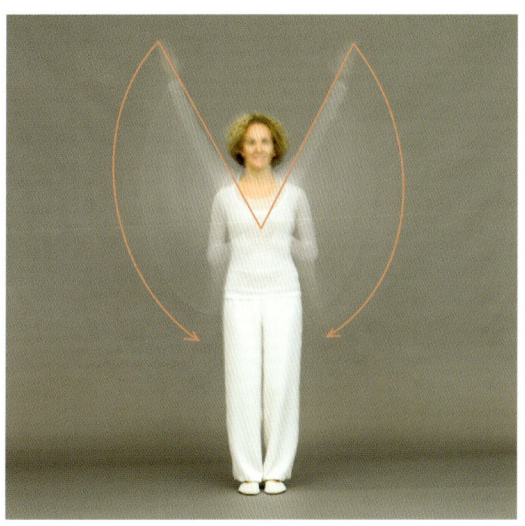 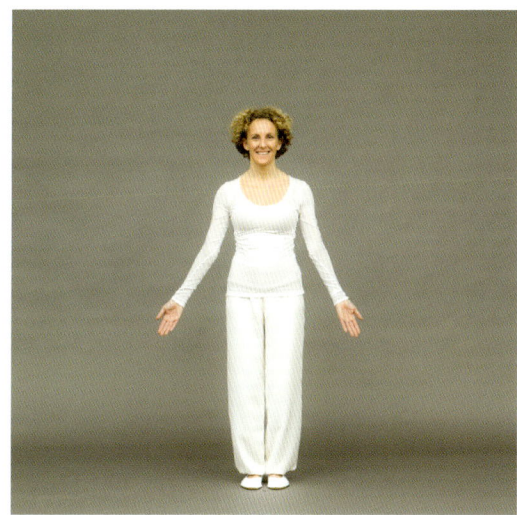

3 Lead the arms downwards in a light, dynamic movement that begins from the shoulder blades. Let them slowly sink down, and feel the movement reaching all the way down to your feet.

4 Release with your arms out by your sides.

Soul Exercises

E (eh) Love

- ✺ Encourages breath, warmth, strength
- ✺ Harmonises the cardio-respiratory system
- ✺ Regulates the relationship between your centre and your surroundings

Intention I can open myself lovingly to the world, but can always return to myself again.

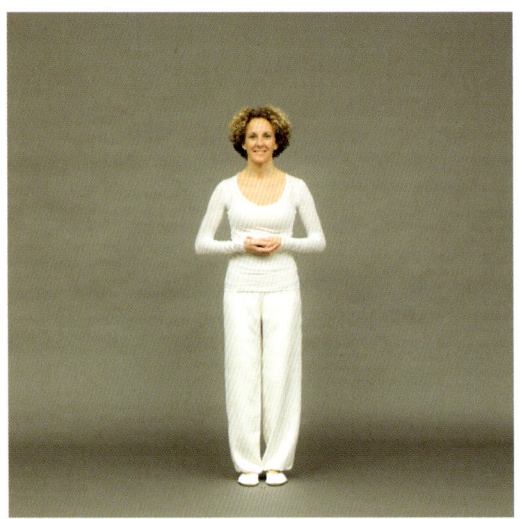 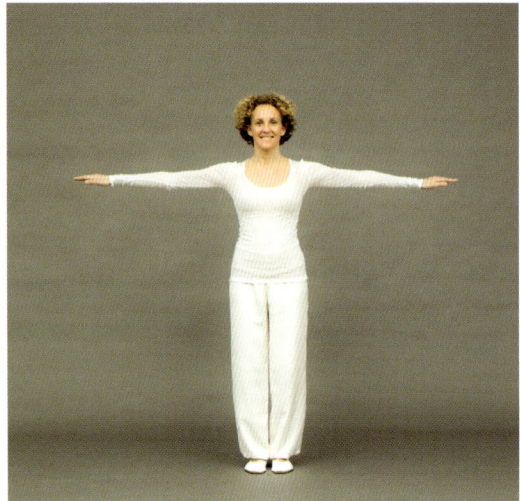

1 Stand upright. Feel a connection to the earth with your feet. Keep your knees loose and breathe calmly. Cup your hands together, level with your diaphragm. Rest your gaze on the horizon. The movement impulse will emanate from your heart.

2 Spread your arms out horizontally, to give a feeling of the broadest possible expansion. Alternatively, the movement can be done in a circular gesture.

Soul Exercises

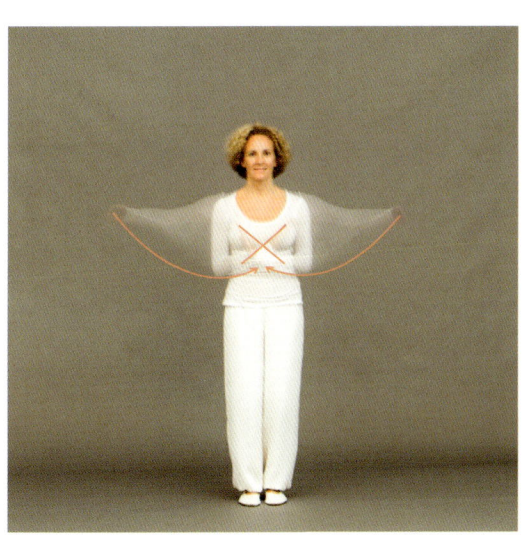 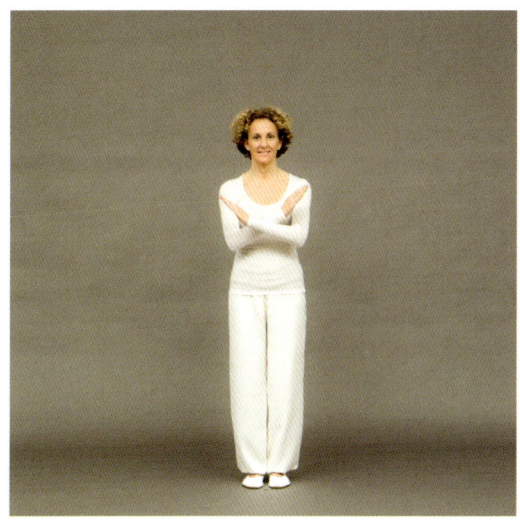

3 Then, gently cross your arms in front of your heart.

4 Release your arms downwards.

Soul Exercises

U (oo) Hope

- ☼ Encourages groundedness, calm, centredness
- ☼ Harmonising the breathing rhythm
- ☼ Warms and strengthens the body

Intention Forming these two wide arcs with my arms, I can send up my hopes and wishes.

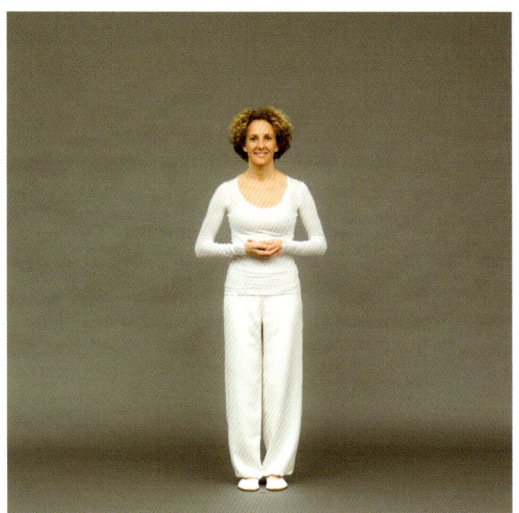 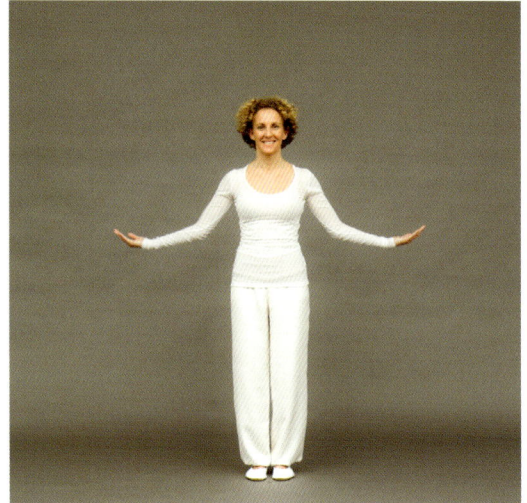

1 Stand upright. Feel a connection to the earth with your feet. Keep your knees loose and breathe calmly. Cup your hands together, level with your diaphragm. Rest your gaze on the horizon. The movement impulse will emanate from your heart.

2 Shift your weight onto your heels and slightly part your toes. On either side of your body, scoop your arms out wide to form two open vessels.

Soul Exercises

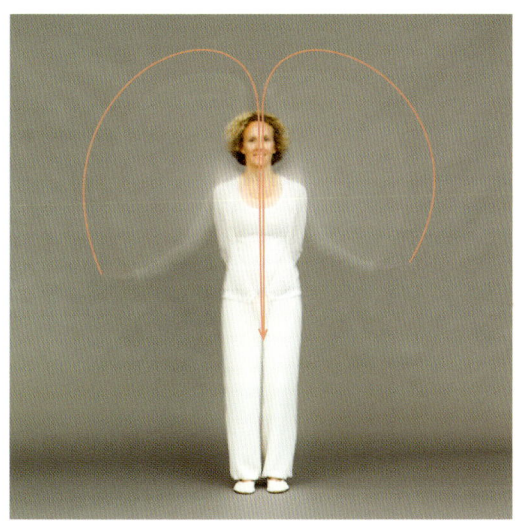

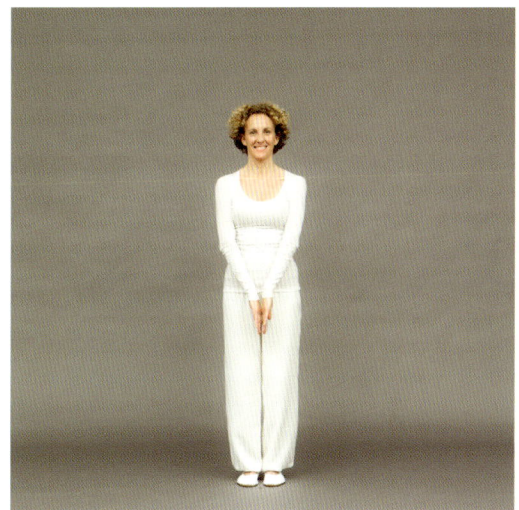

3 Place your feet together and arc your arms over your head until your fingertips meet, pointing downwards. Then lead your hands down in front of you, rising onto your tiptoes, if you wish.

4 Briefly hold this position, then release your arms and heels downwards.

Yes / no

- Encourages structure, harmony, activity
- Strengthens coordination
- Deepens breathing

Intention The forward movement is my affirmation, and the backward movement is my negation.

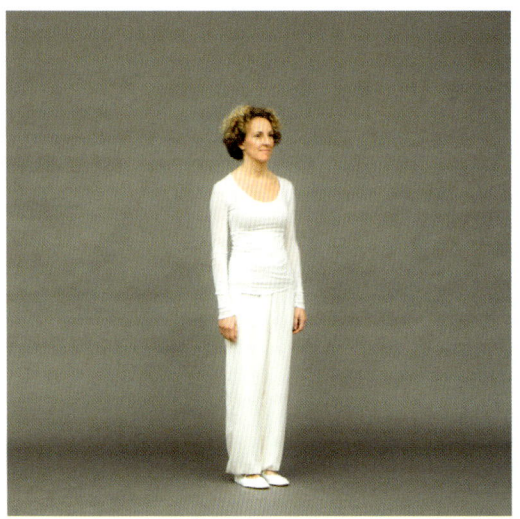 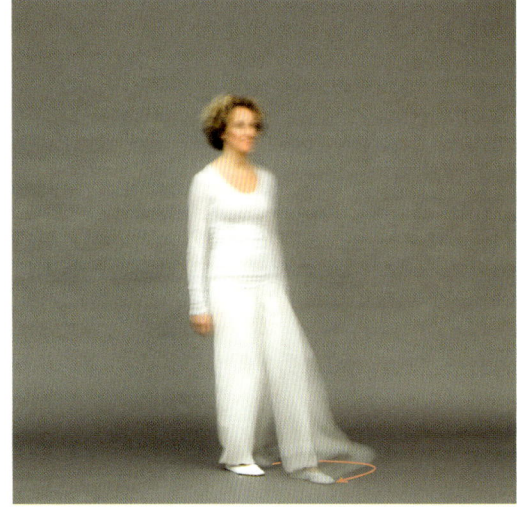

1 Stand upright. Feel a connection to the earth with your feet. Keep your knees loose and breathe calmly. Let your arms hang by your sides. Rest your gaze on the horizon. The movement impulse will emanate from your heart.

2 Move your left foot energetically in a semi-circular curve in front of you. Then place your foot down flat.

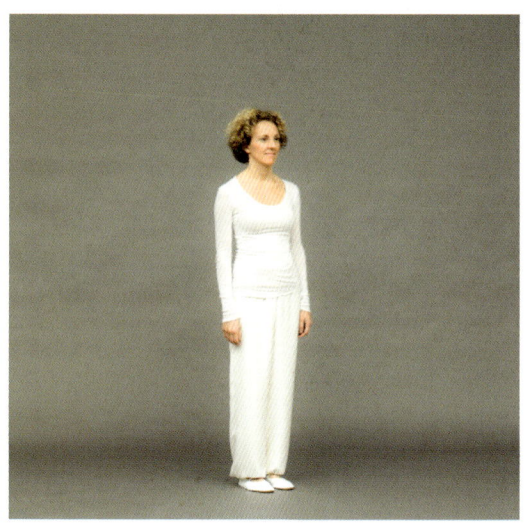 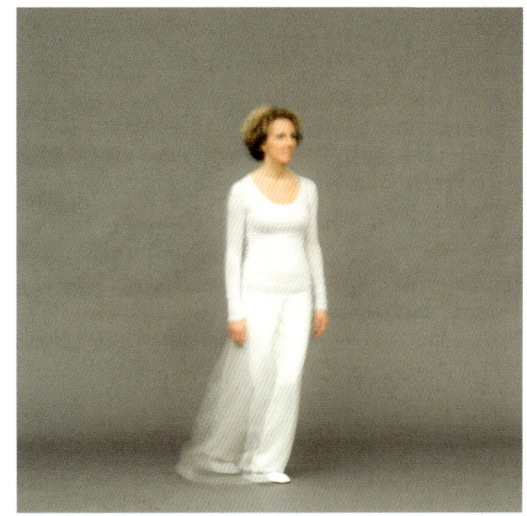

3 Draw the foot back to its starting position.

4 Now move the right foot backwards in a semi-circle, place it down on the ground behind you and draw it forward to the starting position.

Tips

- Repeat this exercise ten times, increasing your speed as you go.
- Whenever one of your feet is set down, briefly rest your weight on both feet equally.

Soul Exercises

Sympathy / antipathy

☼ Encourages balance, connection, stimulation

☼ Aids circulation and digestion

Intention In the forward movement I am sympathetic, accepting and inviting. In the backward movement I am defensive and withdrawing.

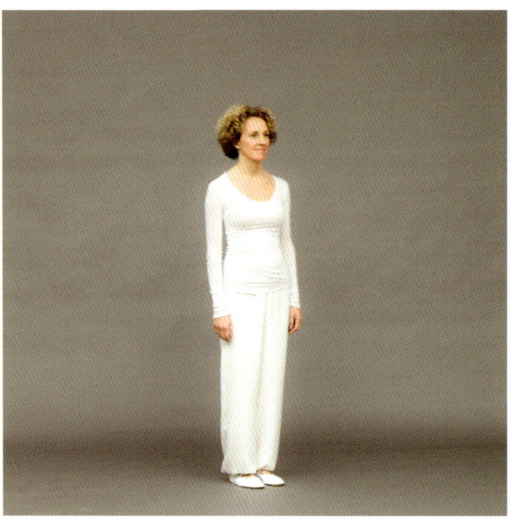 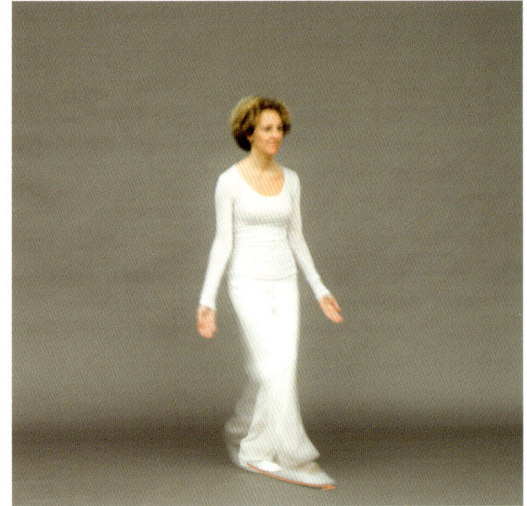

1 Stand upright. Feel a connection to the earth with your feet. Keep your knees loose and breathe calmly. Let your arms hang by your sides. Rest your gaze on the horizon. The movement impulse will emanate from your heart.

2 Feel your way slowly forward with your right foot. Bend your upper body with it in a receiving gesture. Accompany this with open arms, palms facing forward.

Soul Exercises

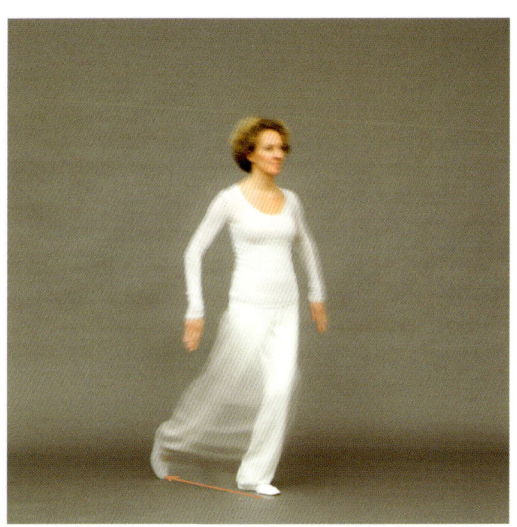

3 Now draw your right foot backwards behind you until your leg is fully extended. You can also move your arms backwards too, palms facing behind you, and hold them in a rejecting gesture.

Tips

✿ Ideally, the right foot will move forwards and backwards without pause.

✿ This exercise should be repeated ten times.

Resources

Where to find a eurythmy therapist

Eurythmy therapy is offered in some Waldorf schools and kindergartens, in clinics, retirement homes, social therapy, at rehab centres and in therapeutic community and curative education settings. It is also available from freelance practitioners all over the world.

Membership of a professional eurythmy therapy association guarantees that its members have undertaken appropriate training, and and gives assurance of quality and standards.

UK

Eurythmy Therapy Association
eurythmytherapyassociation.uk

Council for Anthroposophic Health and Social Care
www.cahsc.org

Europe

International Eurythmy Therapy Forum
heileurythmie-medsektion.net/en

AnthroMed – the Network of Anthroposophical Medicine
www.anthromed.de

Alanus University of Arts and Social Sciences
alanus.edu/eng

USA and Canada

Association for Therapeutic Eurythmy in North America
therapeuticeurythmy.org

Australia and New Zealand

Eurythmy Therapy Association
www.eurythmytherapy.nz

References

Cysarz, Dirk et al. (2004) 'Oscillations of heart rate and respiration synchronise during poetry recitation', in: *American Journal of Physiology – Heart and Circulatory Physiology*, 287:2.

Condon, Willian S. and Louis W. Sander (1974) 'Synchrony demonstrated between movements of the neonate and adult speech', in: *Child Development*, 45:2, 456–462.

Gómez, Milán et al. (2013) 'The Kiki-Bouba effect: A case of personification and ideaesthesia' in *The Journal of Consciousness Studies*. 20:1.2, 84–102.

Further reading

Bryer, Estelle: *Movement for the Young Child*, Waldorf Early Childhood Association North America, USA

Husemann, Armin J.: *Harmony of the Human Body*, Floris Books

Husemann, Armin J.: *Human Hearing and the Reality of Music*, USA: Steiner Books, 2013.

Kirchner-Bockholt, Maragrete: *Foundations of Creative Eurythmy*, Floris Books

Laue, Hans-Broder and Elke E. von: *Physiology of Eurythmy Therapy*, Floris Books

Maintier, Serge: *Speech – Invisible Creation in the Air: Vortices and the Enigma of Speech Sounds*, New York: SteinerBooks, 2016.

Poplawski, Thomas: *Eurythmy: A Short Introduction to the Art of Movement*, Floris Books

Powell, Robert: *Cultivating Inner Radiance and the Body of Immortality*, Lindisfarne Books

Russell, Leonore: *Kinesthetic Learning for Adolescents*, Waldorf Publications, USA

Steiner, Rudolf, GA 277a: *Eurythmy: Its Birth and Development*

Acknowledgements

We wish to thank the Institute for Eurythmy Therapy at Alanus University for making this book possible; our funders for their financial support; and Futurum Verlag for its committed support to the project.

I would also like to thank patients at Casa di Salute Raphael, without whose questions the idea for this book would not have arisen. And Dr Stefano Gasperi, Dr Vinceno Bertozzi and Dr Elfriede Egger, who accompanied the book's development and offered helpful advice.

My personal thanks, too, to Alex, Evi, Nadja, Angelus, Anna, Georg, Claudia and Nelly.

Barbara Tapfer

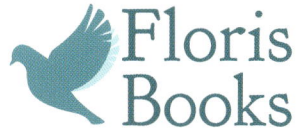
Floris Books

For news on all the latest books, and exclusive discounts, join our mailing list at:

florisbooks.co.uk/mail/

And get a FREE book
with every online order!

We will never pass your details to anyone else.